THE LIFE AND DEATH OF RYAN WHITE

GENDER AND AMERICAN CULTURE

The Gender and American Culture series, guided by feminist perspectives, examines the social construction and influence of gender and sexuality within the full range of American cultures. Books in the series explore the intersection of gender with such markers of difference as race, class, and region. The series presents outstanding scholarship from all areas of American studies—including history, literature, religion, folklore, ethnography, and the visual arts—that investigates in a thoroughly contextualized and lively fashion the ways in which gender works with and against these markers. In so doing, the series seeks to reveal how these complex interactions have shaped American life.

A complete list of books published in Gender and American Culture is available at https://uncpress.org/series/gender-and-american-culture.

THE LIFE AND DEATH OF RYAN WHITE

AIDS AND INEQUALITY IN AMERICA

PAUL M. RENFRO

The University of North Carolina Press | Chapel Hill

Manufactured in the United States of America

Designed by April Leidig
Set in Arnhem by Copperline Book Services

Cover art courtesy Howard County Historical Society, Kokomo, IN.

Library of Congress Cataloging-in-Publication Data
Names: Renfro, Paul M., 1987– author.
Title: The life and death of Ryan White : AIDS and inequality in America / Paul M. Renfro.
Other titles: Gender & American culture.
Description: Chapel Hill : The University of North Carolina Press, [2024] | Series: Gender and American culture | Includes bibliographical references and index.
Identifiers: LCCN 2024023924 | ISBN 9781469680842 (cloth ; alk. paper) | ISBN 9781469680859 (pbk. ; alk. paper) | ISBN 9781469680866 (epub) | ISBN 9781469680873 (pdf)
Subjects: LCSH: White, Ryan. | AIDS (Disease)—Patients—United States—Biography. | AIDS (Disease)—Patients—Public opinion. | AIDS (Disease)—Social aspects—United States. | AIDS (Disease)—Government policy—United States. | BISAC: BIOGRAPHY & AUTOBIOGRAPHY / Medical (incl. Patients) | SOCIAL SCIENCE / Discrimination | LCGFT: Biographies.
Classification: LCC RC606.55.W45 R36 2024 | DDC 362.19697/920092 [B]—dc23/eng/20240613
LC record available at https://lccn.loc.gov/2024023924

For all who have been
touched by HIV and AIDS

CONTENTS

ILLUSTRATIONS

FIGURES

MAPS

ABBREVIATIONS

ACT UP	AIDS Coalition to Unleash Power
AIDS	acquired immunodeficiency syndrome
CARE Act	Ryan White Comprehensive AIDS Resources Emergency Act (1990)
CDC	Centers for Disease Control (later Centers for Disease Control and Prevention)
DNC	Democratic National Convention
FDA	Food and Drug Administration
HIV	human immunodeficiency virus
IDOE	Indiana Department of Education
ISBH	Indiana State Board of Health
LGBTQ+	lesbian, gay, bisexual, trans*, queer, and plus
MSM	men who have/had sex with men
NHF	National Hemophilia Foundation
PCP	Pneumocystis carinii pneumonia
PWA/S	person/people with AIDS
WMS	Western Middle School
WSC	Western School Corporation

A NOTE ON TERMINOLOGY

The words we use matter, especially when writing about complex and sensitive topics such as HIV/AIDS. Activist and writer Michael Callen (1956–93) went so far as to call AIDS a "linguistic battlefield." Thus, a brief note on terminology is in order. Although researchers settled on the term "HIV" in 1986, it is used throughout this book, sometimes anachronistically, for the sake of consistency. Certain problematic terms and phrases—such as "innocent" or "normal"—occasionally appear without quotation marks. Finally, because some people with hemophilia and their allies object to the term "hemophiliac," it is used here only when it appears in quoted source material or in references to the so-called 4-Hs, the four "risk groups" initially associated with HIV/AIDS (homosexuals, hemophiliacs, heroin users, and Haitians). My thanks go to historian Ruth Reichard for her guidance on this last point.

THE LIFE AND DEATH OF RYAN WHITE

INTRODUCTION

Another drug-user, another homosexual, another sex-worker: their contraction of HIV is not newsworthy—there is simply nothing to tell the public about people with AIDS until it appears in some venue thought immune to it.

Thomas Yingling, "Wittgenstein's Tumor," 1992

In the late 1980s, the artist collective Gran Fury, which grew out of the AIDS Coalition to Unleash Power (ACT UP), began spreading a succinct yet powerful message: *All People with AIDS Are Innocent*.[1] This declaration came in response to the widespread cultural embrace of presumably innocent people with AIDS (PWAs) and the simultaneous demonization of other groups that were disproportionately affected by HIV and AIDS—namely gay men, women, trans people, and those who used intravenous drugs. For the members of Gran Fury, distinguishing between "innocent" and "less innocent" PWAs implied "that some people are more deserving of AIDS than others," writes Jack Lowery, "which was anathema to ACT UP's notion that people with AIDS deserve healthcare, not blame."[2] Through its clear and inclusive declaration, Gran Fury implored the public to reject entrenched stigmas regarding certain modes of HIV transmission—and thus to reject a narrow, exclusionary vision of innocence.

No one embodied this vision of innocence more than Ryan White. Born on December 6, 1971, and diagnosed with severe hemophilia shortly thereafter, Ryan Wayne White contracted HIV through contaminated blood products in the early 1980s, and he was diagnosed with AIDS in December 1984. Ryan became a household name in 1985 after he was barred from attending his middle school in Russiaville, Indiana, a suburb of Kokomo, on account of his condition. Even though medical professionals had determined, by that point, that HIV spread primarily through certain sexual activities, needle-sharing, blood products, and blood transfusions—not through casual

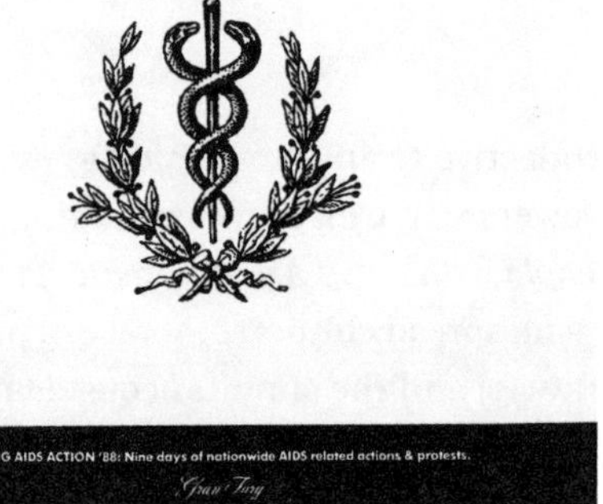

Gran Fury, *All People with AIDS Are Innocent*, 1988. Whitney Museum of American Art, New York City. Gift of Gran Fury.

contact—local parents and school administrators feared White and sought to keep him out of area schools. Across the country, hundreds of other school-age children and adolescents living with HIV/AIDS encountered hostile administrators, parents, and fellow students, but White's case generated unprecedented news media and political attention.[3]

As Ryan achieved a curious kind of stardom in the mid- to late 1980s, his story became a fulcrum around which public perceptions of HIV and AIDS shifted. National news media coverage of Ryan's saga, which spotlighted the efforts of his family and his attorneys to affirm his right to attend school, forced the American public to reckon with prevailing misconceptions about the AIDS epidemic. By introducing Americans to a PWA who was young, white, midwestern, heterosexual, middle-class, photogenic, "normal," and "innocent," media narratives helped undermine reigning ideas of HIV/AIDS as solely a "gay plague" or an illness for "junkies."

Yet for all that White's story did to complicate dominant conceptions of HIV/AIDS, it also reinforced existing hierarchies and prejudices. By distinguishing Ryan from those who contracted HIV through sex or intravenous drug use, media accounts hardened the boundary between "innocent" and "guilty" individuals living with AIDS. "I think it's sad that he had to catch AIDS," one of his schoolmates asserted in a 1985 *NBC Nightly News* broadcast, "because it's not his fault." In 1987, members of the *Indianapolis Star* editorial board cautioned, "It is not the Ryan Whites, the innocents who contracted the disease through blood transfusions, [that] the state must guard against." Rather, they insisted, "health officials must be wary of . . . the AIDS-carriers who don't give a hoot about whether they infect other people, who refuse to change their promiscuous lifestyles and refuse to take precautions." As a "poster child" of sorts, Ryan White taught policymakers and the general public that even "innocents" could contract HIV/AIDS, and he therefore "helped to humanize AIDS," as one Presbyterian minister put it.[4]

White's "innocence" and "humanity" required the opposing forces of guilt and inhumanity.[5] These forces would appear, first and foremost, in the queer people, drug users, and other stigmatized populations who supposedly "refuse[d] to take precautions" against HIV/AIDS. But guilt and inhumanity would also be found in the individuals and communities who shunned PWAs. In that vein, Ryan White and his story provided grist for what scholar Cindy Patton calls the "national pedagogy" on AIDS.[6] This widely disseminated set of "lessons" stressed tolerance and awareness yet clearly differentiated between "at-risk" and "safe" populations, thereby bolstering already powerful stigmas and obscuring the structural and systemic factors that fueled the HIV/AIDS epidemic—particularly homophobia, racism, sexism, poverty, and uneven access to health care.

Residents of Kokomo and surrounding communities emerged as major villains in the Ryan White saga and as prime examples of intolerance and cruelty in the national pedagogy on AIDS. National news media stories and a 1989 ABC made-for-television movie blamed Ryan's troubles on Kokomo and its poor and working-class white community. If Ryan's neighbors could simply treat him with respect and kindness and allow him to attend school, the prevailing narrative went, then all would be well. This narrative and the broader national pedagogy in which it fit were cynically appropriated by none other than President Ronald Reagan, whose inadequate response to the epidemic exacerbated the stigmas surrounding HIV/AIDS

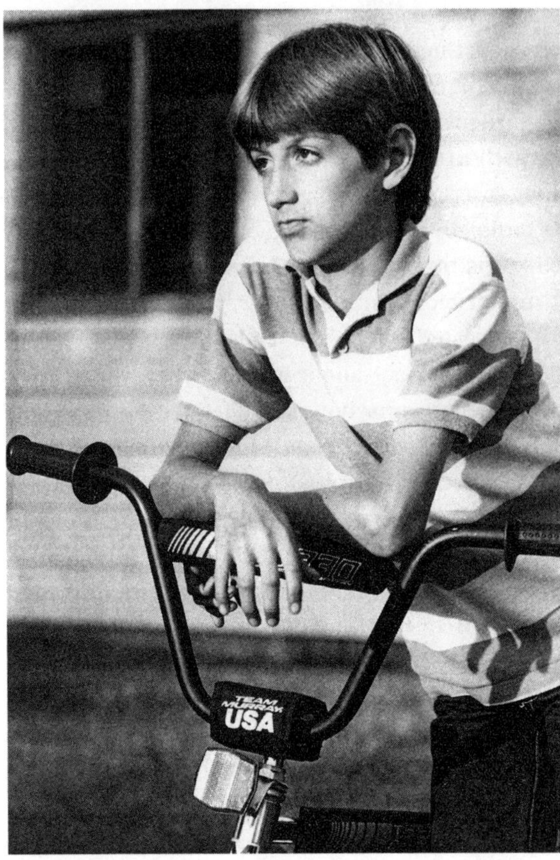

Ryan White leans on the handlebars of his bicycle, circa 1985. Howard County Historical Society, Kokomo, IN.

and cost thousands upon thousands of lives. Reagan's obituary for White, published in the *Washington Post*, urged Americans "to be compassionate, caring and tolerant toward those with AIDS."[7] By concentrating on the harassment that Ryan White endured in the Kokomo area, then, journalists, politicians, and other observers could reduce a structural, global crisis to an interpersonal one.[8]

Because Ryan White was arguably the world's most famous PWA at the time of his death in April 1990, his passing was a major event. Held at the cavernous Second Presbyterian Church in the affluent Indianapolis neighborhood of Meridian Hills, Ryan's funeral attracted over 1,500 mourners—including First Lady Barbara Bush, Indiana governor Evan Bayh, Michael Jackson, and Elton John, who performed a rendition of his song "Skyline Pigeon" at the ceremony. While Ronald Reagan's obituary for Ryan insisted that "there have been too many funerals like his," hardly any funerals resembled Ryan White's.[9] Many other AIDS deaths were barely marked at all, a fact that spurred one ACT UP affinity group to stage "political funerals" in the years after Ryan's death. These actions served as poignant critiques of the state and societal neglect endured by so many PWAs and their extended kinship networks.

Such militant, confrontational activism had become more and more common beginning in the mid- to late 1980s, just as Ryan became a household name. While anger and rage were conspicuously absent from Ryan's advocacy and personal story, activists affiliated with ACT UP and other groups increasingly expressed their frustration in the face of organized abandonment.[10] Ostracized in a way that Ryan White never would be, ACT UP members and similarly minded activists rejected respectability politics and what political scientist Cathy Cohen calls "secondary marginalization," the process by which subjugated groups petition for citizenship rights and improved social standing by deserting their most vulnerable members.[11] This kind of radical AIDS activism unfolded alongside and occasionally in indirect opposition to certain versions of the Ryan White story—namely those that celebrated Ryan while ignoring or even denigrating other PWAs.

In the wake of Ryan's highly publicized death, however, many AIDS activists begrudgingly supported the US Congress's decision to name a major AIDS relief package after the young man—rather than after another, perhaps more representative, person with AIDS. The Ryan White Comprehensive AIDS Resources Emergency (CARE) Act helped deliver much-needed federal funding for HIV/AIDS prevention and treatment, yet it also intensified AIDS-related stigmas and reified hierarchies of victimhood "that placed innocent children above implicitly guilty homosexuals."[12] Although the use of "a politically safe symbol" (in one reporter's words) may have guaranteed the passage of the CARE Act, it also placed profound limits on the scope and scale of the legislation and the programs it created.[13] Not only did the Ryan White CARE Act fail to address the underlying causes of the epidemic, but it also contained draconian amendments barring the use of federal funds for needle-exchange programs and sex education. These sorts of measures proved disproportionately harmful to queer people and people of color. Furthermore, funding issues plagued the CARE Act throughout the 1990s.

With the growing availability of protease inhibitors and highly active antiretroviral therapy in the mid- to late 1990s—for those with access to decent health care, that is—a "general sense that AIDS is over" took hold among a broad swath of the American population.[14] The late 1990s and first decade of the 2000s also witnessed the increasing "globalization of AIDS," through which Americans increasingly came to believe that HIV/AIDS existed primarily (if not exclusively) in the Global South, namely Africa. Since the consolidation of the highly active antiretroviral therapy regime and the globalization of AIDS, the dominant cultural narratives concerning HIV and AIDS have therefore centered on the presumed "end of AIDS" or "AIDS obsolescence," as Jih-Fei Cheng, Alexandra Juhasz, and Nishant Shahani have documented.[15] "For people with insurance, stable housing, and individualized support," scholar and activist Ted Kerr explains, "HIV can be a manageable chronic illness, a situation between patient and doctor. For people who have been minoritized and are without economic stability, HIV exacerbates preexisting crises, which often are dealt with less by friends and lovers and more by social workers, and increasingly by the criminal justice system."[16] Ryan White's story, which includes the passage of the CARE Act in 1990, helped lay the groundwork for narratives of AIDS obsolescence. As Leonard Calabrese, the cochair of the AIDS Commission of Greater Cleveland, noted after Ryan's death in 1990, "America is a funny country. We seem to focus so intensely on a problem for a brief period of time and then move on to other things. We've done that with AIDS." Yet despite the allure of the "end of AIDS" narrative, "the AIDS story isn't over," Calebrese asserted.[17] HIV and AIDS would continue to ravage communities of color in the United States and globally long after Ryan's demise.[18]

The Ryan White saga is also fundamentally about whiteness, then.[19] While journalists, politicians, and other commentators rarely mentioned Ryan White's race, they didn't have to. In the narratives they wove about Ryan's life and death, his youth, innocence, and normality often stood in for or silently buttressed his whiteness. Moreover, Ryan White's very public life and death both reflected and shaped a broader cultural and political fixation on white male PWAs. As Cheng, Juhasz, and Shahani argue, "cisgender white gay men" have long served as "the primary default setting for academic theorizations, public health and medical initiatives, and popular culture revisitations" of AIDS.[20] Although Ryan White proved that AIDS wasn't simply the "*gay* white man's disease" that many imagined it to be, his story suggested to Americans that AIDS was still a disease of white males.[21] This wasn't true, of course, as Black and Brown people bore the brunt of the epidemic during Ryan's life and after his death, and women and their children often faced AIDS without any formal recognition or support. (Until 1993, the Centers for Disease Control and Prevention effectively excluded women from its case definition of AIDS.) Ryan White overshadowed these other populations living with, and dying from, HIV/AIDS—including similarly "innocent" Black and Brown children, many of whom had contracted HIV from their mothers during childbirth. As the Black newsmagazine *Emerge* noted in 1990, the year Ryan died, 52 percent of children living with AIDS in the United States were Black.[22]

Narratives of AIDS obsolescence are thus narratives of erasure. Some critics may claim that this book replicates such narratives by centering an "innocent" white male with AIDS. But in keeping with the tradition of critical whiteness studies, *The Life and Death of Ryan White* seeks to interrogate dominant ideologies and narratives in order to unsettle them. Accordingly, readers should come away with a deeper understanding of how HIV and AIDS affected women and people of color before, during, and after Ryan's battle with AIDS. On that score, this book illustrates how public interest in HIV/AIDS began to wane as white Americans became less susceptible to infection and serious complications. "There was a white epidemic, and there is an African American, person of color epidemic," HIV/AIDS activist Dr. Bambi Gaddist observed in 2017. "There was an interest when it was a white epidemic. But somehow over these past thirty years, as it's changed its face, there's a lack of discussion and interest."[23] The Ryan White story helped enable this shift by permitting the public to relegate AIDS stigma, AIDS discrimination, and AIDS itself to the past. Yet AIDS stigma, AIDS discrimination, and AIDS persist.

Equipped with this knowledge that "the AIDS crisis is not over," scholars have become increasingly invested in the study of HIV/AIDS over the past decade or so, part of a broader turn toward examining the 1980s, 1990s, and their afterlives.[24] For example, the flagship journal in US history, the *Journal of American History*, published its first "feature-length" piece on HIV/AIDS in 2017.[25] Nonetheless, relatively little has been written about Ryan White.[26] In a similar vein, the CARE Act has received short shrift in the burgeoning literature on HIV/AIDS, and as Cindy Patton notes, few scholars have concentrated on children and childhood within the epidemic.[27] By situating Ryan White within the broader HIV/AIDS epidemic of the 1980s and 1990s, this book demonstrates how racialized notions of childhood innocence and exceptional victimhood shaped understandings of and responses to the crisis.

The Life and Death of Ryan White begins by showing how a slight Indiana youngster with hemophilia became infected with HIV in the early 1980s and emerged as the "innocent" face of the AIDS epidemic in 1985. Chapter 1 traces how the virus that would become known as HIV found its way into the blood supply and eventually into the body of Ryan White. It also illustrates how Ryan's "normality" influenced his relationship to hemophilia and then AIDS, which in turn influenced the public's relationship to and interest in Ryan's story. More specifically, Ryan's whiteness, youth, heterosexuality, and conscious rejection of disability and "otherness" conspired to make him a sympathetic PWA.

The next chapter concentrates on Ryan's highly publicized fight to return to Western Middle School in 1985 and 1986. Even though the risk of transmitting HIV in a typical school setting was and remains virtually nonexistent, school officials prohibited Ryan from attending classes in person because he had AIDS. Attending school was central to Ryan's self-identification as a "normal" child, and the fact that some administrators and concerned parents sought to deprive him of that experience only boosted his public profile and imbued his struggle to go back to school with greater significance. Not only was Ryan battling to return to Western Middle School; he was waging a larger campaign *against* ignorance and fear and *for* education, broadly conceived. This campaign would bolster the national pedagogy on AIDS and help cement Ryan's status as an international celebrity.

Chapter 3 considers Ryan White's growing fame alongside his struggle to return to school. Because his fight to attend school resonated with so many people, and because he did not belong to any of the marginalized groups with which AIDS was most closely associated, Ryan became the (unrepresentative) "poster boy" of the epidemic. His tremendous popularity—augmented, in part, by his friendships with megastars like Elton John and Michael Jackson—enhanced the appeal of the national pedagogy while also drawing attention away from the populations most deeply affected by HIV/AIDS, especially people of color and queer people.

The fourth chapter analyzes the ABC television movie based on Ryan's battle to return to Western Middle School. First broadcast in early 1989, *The Ryan White Story* blames Ryan's plight not on the "blood business" that allowed him to become infected with HIV or on the politicians who failed to limit the scope and severity of the epidemic.[28] Rather, the film pinpoints local townspeople—who are coded as poor and working class—as the primary obstacles to Ryan's happiness and personal fulfillment. *The Ryan White Story* therefore reflected and reinforced Ryan's status as a celebrity and contributed mightily to the national pedagogy, identifying awareness and kindness as potential solutions to the AIDS epidemic while portraying homophobia and ignorance as hallmarks of the white working class.

Just a year after *The Ryan White Story* first aired, its main subject was nearing the end of his miraculous life. Ryan had defied the odds and lived for over five years following his AIDS diagnosis in December 1984. Chapter 5 looks at Ryan's highly publicized death and funeral in April 1990. While many AIDS deaths were concealed or ignored altogether, news media outlets from around the globe covered Ryan's death and funeral, and mourners from far and wide flocked to Indianapolis to pay their respects. Others mailed heartfelt condolences to the White family. In the years after Ryan's high-profile funeral—which was held in a massive Indianapolis church and broadcast live on CNN—AIDS activists demanded the same respect and recognition that had been conferred upon this famous Indiana teenager. Thus, the political funerals they organized not only challenged the state and society to treat all PWAs with dignity, humanity, and care but also exposed the symbolic distance that separated Ryan from other people with HIV/AIDS.

Chapters 6 and 7 show how Ryan's death and funeral set the stage for the Ryan White Comprehensive AIDS Resources Emergency Act, passed and signed into law shortly after he died. Though it represented a significant bipartisan legislative achievement, the CARE Act nevertheless reaffirmed the hierarchies that structured the 1980s and 1990s AIDS epidemic by further elevating an "innocent" PWA and exacerbating the stigmas attached to intravenous drug use and particular sexual behaviors. The CARE Act's funding issues, which spanned Republican and Democratic presidential administrations and periods of congressional rule, also revealed the limits of respectability politics within the AIDS crisis.

Finally, the epilogue considers what Ryan White might mean in the third decade of the twenty-first century, as the world grapples with several interlocking epidemiological crises. In particular, COVID-19 and the mpox virus continue to cause unimaginable grief and suffering the world over. In this context, the story of Ryan White offers both horror and hope. Of course, there is no single Ryan White story but rather thousands of stories deployed for myriad purposes—in the service of exclusion and inclusion, blame and absolution, division and unity. We have similarly crafted countless narratives over the past several years to make sense of COVID-19 and the mpox virus, both of which resemble AIDS in more ways than one.

In the HIV/AIDS, coronavirus, and mpox crises, seductive and pernicious hierarchies of victimhood have emerged, positioning the innocent over the guilty, the clean over the contaminated. Narratives advocating perseverance, personal responsibility, and enlightenment—and obscuring the structural forces that make some populations especially vulnerable to infection, serious illness, and death—have justified a range of health outcomes within these different pandemics.[29] Just as certain populations have been deemed responsible for acquiring (and spreading) HIV and the mpox virus, especially queer people, similarly marginalized groups—from low-wage retail and service workers to the uninsured, from Asian Americans and Jews to the unhoused—have been vilified or rendered disposable during the COVID-19 pandemic. And just as the powerful and well-connected prematurely declared the end of AIDS in the mid-1990s, President Joe Biden told a national television audience in September 2022, "The pandemic is over." Over 12,000 Americans died of COVID that month.[30] Likewise, while predominantly white, cisgender gay men celebrated victory over the mpox virus in 2022 and 2023 following successful yet narrowly focused awareness and vaccination campaigns, they have ignored mpox's disproportionate impact on communities of color in the United States and abroad.[31]

The Ryan White story has similarly been used to draw lines between the beginning and the end, the righteous and the unrighteous, the immune and the vulnerable, and the informed and the ignorant. But it might also help obliterate those boundaries. Ryan's story could be a story about courage in the face of adversity, about the universal search for security and belonging, about love and care within and beyond the bonds of blood, and about what we owe each other. This is Ryan's story.

CHAPTER ONE

BLOOD AND BLAME

It is easy to start an AIDS panic.

Cindy Patton, "Fear of AIDS: The Erotics of Innocence and Ingenuity," 1992

Jeanne White had been in labor for nearly twenty-three hours at Kokomo's St. Joseph Memorial Hospital. After almost a full day of pain and anguish, she finally gave birth to her first child, Ryan Wayne White, on December 6, 1971. But even after she delivered Ryan, named for actor Ryan O'Neal, her "pain didn't stop," Jeanne (pronounced "JEEN-ee") later recalled. "I felt like I was still in labor." She bled profusely and lost consciousness. Doctors "sent helicopters all over Indiana to bring back Rh-negative blood" for her—some thirteen pints overall. Jeanne White's experience mirrored that of her newborn son, who bled incessantly following his circumcision. After the procedure, Ryan was transported to Methodist Hospital in Indianapolis, where a hematologist diagnosed him with classic or severe hemophilia. Although Jeanne's mother and grandmother had tested negative for the hemophilia gene, "the gene just showed up out of the blue, without any inherited tendency."[1]

Ryan's peculiar status in the world of AIDS originated in his struggle with hemophilia. As much as White's severe hemophilia (hemophilia A or classic hemophilia) inhibited him from playing sports or partaking in other activities, his race, class, and heterosexuality enabled him to seem at least somewhat "normal," a status Ryan coveted. "All I ever wanted to do was be one of the kids," he shared in his coauthored (and posthumously published) autobiography.[2] The advent and growing accessibility of blood-clotting products over the first decade of Ryan's life facilitated this pursuit of "normality" by allowing him to ride his bicycle and engage in other potentially dangerous activities. Yet these sorts of products, namely Factor VIII, would also lead to his HIV infection and subsequent AIDS diagnosis. The blood products industry could have done much more to ensure the safety of such products, but it failed to do so. As a result, thousands upon thousands of people with hemophilia fell ill, including Ryan White. Yet the "blood business" generally avoided the blame and scorn heaped upon gay men and people who used intravenous drugs during the early years of the HIV/AIDS epidemic.

When Ryan was diagnosed with AIDS in December 1984, it complicated his pursuit of "normality." But Ryan's identity markers—as a white, midwestern, middle-class, cisgender, superficially able-bodied teenager—in addition to the fact that he acquired HIV "through no fault of his own" (as many saw it), distinguished him from other PWAs and other people with disabilities.[3] Further, even after his AIDS diagnosis, Ryan sought to obscure both his hemophilia and AIDS, a posture enabled by sympathetic news media accounts that stressed the boy's "normality." "Let's just pretend I don't have it," he famously told his mother.[4]

Before Ryan White's AIDS diagnosis, white gay men in certain urban areas represented "the first visible group of people dying of AIDS."[5] Many observers therefore understood HIV/AIDS as a "gay plague" in the early 1980s and beyond. Accordingly, when medical researchers learned of people with hemophilia contracting HIV through contaminated blood products, gay men emerged as scapegoats. Despite AIDS activists' efforts to highlight the fact that "anyone is vulnerable to infection," the idea that HIV was "spreading" from gay men to the "general population" proved difficult to shake.[6] Similarly, the distinction between "guilty" people with AIDS (who were responsible for their fate) and "innocent" PWAs (who had been stricken with HIV/AIDS "through no fault of [their] own") also loomed over the Ryan White saga, shaping news media and public interest in his case. Ultimately, White's hemophilia—along with his race, age, heterosexuality, and "innocence"—helped make him a vulnerable and sympathetic "AIDS victim," one who could conceivably assimilate into mainstream, "normal" society.[7]

HOPE AND HAZARD

Hemophilia is a rare, often-inherited bleeding disorder that primarily affects males. It prevents the efficient clotting of blood, meaning that those with hemophilia bleed excessively and sometimes unexpectedly. They also bruise easily and frequently experience pain and swelling in their joints. The earliest known mention of hemophilia appears in the Babylonian Talmud, which dates back to around 200 CE. But formal scientific and medical management of the disease began in earnest in the nineteenth century. It was then, historian Stephen Pemberton details, that hemophilia "became an object of continuous medical and scientific concern." Nineteenth-century efforts to understand and treat the disorder set the stage for profound research and treatment advancements in the twentieth century. Developments in the fields of coagulation, blood storage, and transfusion around the turn of the century would significantly improve the life chances of children born with hemophilia in the World War II era and beyond. By the end of the Second World War, blood and plasma transfusions had become "routine" and "relatively safe," even though hemophilia remained a dismal, painful, and highly lethal disease into the 1950s.[8]

Still, the immediate postwar years held tremendous promise for people with hemophilia and their families—not only in the medical and scientific realms but also with respect to the formation of a discrete, organized community. As Susan Resnik notes, 1948 was "a defining year for hemophilia." It marked the beginning of a fruitful decade for coagulation research (1948–58) and saw the establishment of the Hemophilia Foundation. Later renamed the National Hemophilia Foundation (NHF), the group would formalize and strengthen the bonds between people with hemophilia across the United States and advocate on their behalf in the halls of power. Further, the coagulation research undertaken during this ten-year period led to the discovery of cryoprecipitate—"a cold precipitate of plasma" that "contained a high concentration of clotting material (AHF, or Factor VIII)"—as a treatment for bleeding episodes. Though celebrated as a "medical milestone," cryoprecipitate took considerable time to administer and "required special refrigeration," thus precluding at-home use. Its discovery nevertheless helped inaugurate a "golden era" for hemophilia research and treatment, paving the way for the development of easily accessible concentrates.[9]

Ryan White was born in this "golden era" for research and treatment. Factor VIII and other products that promoted clotting became more widely available in the 1960s and 1970s. These treatments could be administered at home or on the go, so those with hemophilia could avoid onerous trips to the hospital in the event of a bleeding episode. As one 1983 article in Cleveland's *Plain Dealer* indicated, these advances "revolutionized the lives of hemophiliacs. No longer must a bleed mean several days in the hospital" or "several hours in an emergency room."[10] In this same moment, the NHF increasingly functioned as a political advocacy organization, in much the same way that the American Diabetes Association did. With more and more people with hemophilia gaining access to home therapies such as Factor VIII, some observers compared their circumstances to those of diabetics, whose self-administered injections of insulin offered them autonomy

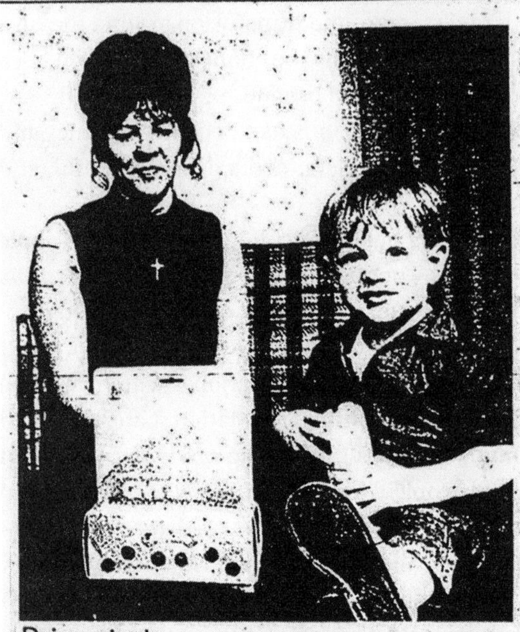
THE KOKOMO TRIBUNE

Page 2 SATURDAY, MARCH 17, 1973

Drive starts

Ryan White, poster boy for the Howard County Hemophilia Society, inspects a donation box for the society's 1973 fund drive which begins today. Looking on is Mrs. C. E. Dietzen, campaign chairman. Volunteer workers will conduct the door-to-door campaign until March 24 and a benefit basketball game will be held March 29 in the gymnasium of St. Patrick Parochial School. (Tribune photo)

Ryan White as a "poster boy" for hemophilia. *Kokomo Tribune*, March 17, 1973.

and improved their standard of living. The NHF and the American Diabetes Association also undertook similar lobbying efforts in this period to secure funding and guarantees of medical coverage.[11]

In the 1970s and beyond, people with hemophilia and diabetes both grappled with questions of ability and normality, which would loom large in the Ryan White saga. The growing visibility of the disability rights movement during the 1970s forced people with diabetes and people with hemophilia to determine "whether or not to be considered under the rubric of 'the handicapped,'" Resnik writes. This "philosophical dilemma" would arise in the courtroom battles waged over Ryan's right to return to school in Howard County, as the White family attorneys flirted with the idea of positioning Ryan "as a special-education student."[12] For their part, the Whites often affirmed Ryan's ability despite the challenges he faced. "Kids don't talk to him like he's retarded," Ryan's mother, Jeanne, told *People* magazine in 1988. "I wonder why adults do? Ryan can't figure it out."[13]

As liberating as Factor VIII and other self-administered treatments may have been for those with hemophilia in the "golden era," some of these treatments proved riskier than others—even before the 1980s HIV/AIDS epidemic. Jih-Fei Cheng and others have shown how the rapid development and expansion of the American pharmaceutical and global blood biotech industries in the twentieth century enabled the spread of "many viral epidemics and pandemics, including hepatitis C and HIV/AIDS." This industrialization and "commodification of blood"—what Resnik calls the "blood business"—dramatically transformed the lives of people with hemophilia in both positive and negative ways.[14] By the late 1970s, "the development of freeze-dried blood-clotting factors drawn from multiple donors" meant that "hemophiliacs could infuse themselves at home, giving them a freedom that they had not enjoyed before."[15] Yet this new reality presented new perils, as well. Whereas each bag of cryoprecipitate included material from just one donor, Factor VIII and other concentrates pooled blood and plasma from thousands of donors. Each injection therefore introduced the blood of thousands of people (if not tens of thousands) into a user's body.[16] By 1983, over 80 percent of those with severe hemophilia who had been treated with concentrate showed "serologic evidence of previous exposure to hepatitis B antigen," although many "considered the risk of hepatitis to be an acceptable price to pay for the benefits of AHF concentrate."[17] Ryan White himself tested positive for hepatitis B in November 1984, just before his AIDS diagnosis.[18] As HIV/AIDS spread in the early 1980s—before the pervasive use of heat treatment to eliminate HIV in the blood supply—Factor VIII represented both a "lifeline" and a potential death sentence for people with hemophilia.[19] As one Associated Press story put it, "For many hemophiliacs, AIDS has meant a conscious decision to avoid taking the clotting factor that has so improved their lives in the past decade."[20]

This AP story also reflected the tensions between disability and "normality" that shaped the lives of those with hemophilia like Ryan White. The article included quotations from NHF officials who decried the fact that HIV/AIDS would drive people with hemophilia back to the dark ages, before the advent of Factor VIII. "This is a treatment that has really liberated hemophiliacs from being disabled people," declared Alan Brownstein, then executive director of the NHF. "It is such a crying shame." Charles Carman, chairman of the NHF board and head of the organization's AIDS task force, struck similar notes. "Concentrate was a dream come true," Carman insisted. "It's the difference between having to live a cloistered, protected, low-productivity life and being able to be a normal, productive, tax-paying citizen." Their fusion of ability, liberation, and productivity—and, by implication, of disability, unfreedom, and dependency—served to distance people with hemophilia from people with disabilities. Ryan White's supporters, and occasionally his detractors, would employ similar rhetorical flourishes as they portrayed the Indiana teenager as "normal," a loaded designation that renounced not only disability but also other forms of perceived deviance, such as homosexuality.[21]

"GAY BLOOD, BAD BLOOD"

Almost exactly a year after the *New York Times* announced the discovery of a "rare cancer" in forty-one gay men, activists and medical professionals met at Mount Sinai Hospital and the National Gay Task Force (NGTF) offices in New York City to discuss reports of several people with hemophilia stricken with AIDS.[22] During these two meetings, held on July 13 and 14, 1982 (and described in more detail below), representatives from the National Gay Task Force, the Gay Men's Health Crisis, and other groups investigated the "possible relationship between AID[S] and FACTOR VIII blood" while simultaneously working to combat perceptions of gay men as vectors of disease.[23] By underscoring the fact that HIV/AIDS could (and did) affect a wide array of people—not just gay men—activists hoped to forestall any efforts to blame HIV transmission on the gay community. "A panic over blood agent/AID[S] transmission if linked to gays would probably lead to immediate discrimination," read the minutes from one of these meetings. For these activists, "recent AID[S] developments" related to the discovery of AIDS in three adult males with hemophilia "should guide the focus away from the gay community specifically."[24] Although these and subsequent discussions took place well before Ryan White received his AIDS diagnosis in December 1984—following his longtime use of Factor VIII—they foreshadowed the discussions of "guilt" and "innocence" that would mark the White saga. Specifically, these conversations prefigured the ways in which gays and other marginalized populations would bear the brunt of the blame for the AIDS crisis, particularly as it ravaged "innocent" or "normal" groups (such as people with hemophilia) across the eighties.[25]

By the time these initial meetings took place in July 1982, health officials and the press had already constructed HIV/AIDS as primarily, if not exclusively, a "gay" disease. Subsequent research has determined that HIV/AIDS first appeared in humans in the early twentieth century.[26] But even in 1981 and 1982, it was clear that AIDS affected not only gay men but also intravenous drug users and other populations. Still, the dominant etiological, epidemiological, and cultural frameworks through which experts and laypeople alike first understood AIDS rested on preexisting notions of gay male promiscuity. The "immune overload" or "antigen overload" hypothesis, sociologist Steven Epstein shows, "represented the initial medical frame for understanding the epidemic: the syndrome was essentially linked to gay men, specifically to the 'excesses' of the 'homosexual lifestyle.'" According to proponents of this interpretive model, many gay men, especially those living in urban areas, had overwhelmed their immune systems through their sexual profligacy, acquisition of various sexually transmitted diseases, use of treatments to combat those STDs, and drug abuse. These "lifestyle" choices had supposedly subjected gay men to rare opportunistic infections such as Kaposi's sarcoma and Pneumocystis carinii pneumonia (PCP).[27] Extant, exaggerated ideas of gay male promiscuity thus shaped medical and popular knowledge of the illness in this moment and beyond.

Many physicians, researchers, and journalists even preferred the term "gay-related immune deficiency" over other, perhaps less accusatory labels—at least until May 1982, when the Centers for Disease Control (CDC) formally christened the syndrome "AIDS."[28] The term "gay-related immune deficiency" implied that the disease had originated in gay men and among men who had sex with men (MSM) in the late 1970s and early 1980s.[29] But even as this term fell out of favor, its governing logic lived on through the figure of "Patient Zero" and the predatory, promiscuous, queer "HIV monster."[30] "In the eyes of the straight world," Michael Warner wrote in 1995, "gay still means AIDS; to come out is to come into the epidemic."[31]

Given the close association between HIV/AIDS and homosexuality, two July 1982 editions of the CDC's *Morbidity and Mortality Weekly Report* posed formidable challenges to AIDS activists and their allies. The first, published on July 9, noted the appearance of Kaposi's sarcoma and other opportunistic infections "among Haitians residing in the United States."[32] The second, published on July 16, discussed "three cases of Pneumocystis carinii pneumonia among patients with hemophilia A and without other underlying disease." The individuals in question were "heterosexual males" with no "history of intravenous drug abuse."[33] On one hand, these CDC reports fundamentally undermined conceptions of AIDS as an exclusively "gay disease."[34] On the other, the links initially drawn between AIDS cases and the gay community would prove difficult to sever, meaning that gays could easily be blamed for "infecting" other segments of the population. A *Washington Post* article published on July 16, 1982, reflected this logic by describing AIDS as "a type of immune system breakdown that started among homosexual men." The headline, "Strange Disease Now Spreading to Hemophiliacs," positioned "homosexual men" as the "spreaders." A letter to the editor published eight days later rejected the *Post*'s framing. "The disease did not 'start among homosexual men,' but was first *reported* in subsets of them," the author explained.[35]

The ahistorical notion that AIDS had first appeared in gay men and was "now spreading" to other, less stigmatized groups built on two familiar and potent antigay tropes. First, due to the long-standing pathologization and medicalization of homosexuality in the United States, gay men had long carried the stigma of sickness. Only in 1973, less than a decade before the AIDS crisis erupted, did the American Psychological Association remove homosexuality from its *Diagnostic and Statistical Manual of Mental Disorders*, largely in response to activists' demands. Moreover, despite the gradual decriminalization of sodomy in many states across the 1970s, an ascendant religious right continued to conflate homosexuality with pederasty while maintaining that gay men "must recruit" because they "cannot reproduce."[36] The deep ties between homosexuality and illness, first, and homosexuality and contagion, second, enabled commentators—especially newly emboldened opponents of queer liberation—to cast AIDS as a "gay disease" migrating from an inherently deviant and sickly group toward "innocent," healthy, and unsuspecting populations.[37]

Before the CDC released the *Morbidity and Mortality Weekly Report* on hemophilia and AIDS, Dr. James Curran—head of the CDC's AIDS task force—convened representatives from the National Gay Task Force, the Gay Men's Health Crisis, and other groups on July 13, 1982, for the first of the two meetings mentioned earlier. Curran had "called [the] meeting of gay political/health care workers to suggest representation of [the] gay community at the Expert Committee," a panel on AIDS set to meet in Washington, DC, later that month. The Expert Committee included representatives from the CDC, the National Institutes of Health, the American Red Cross, and the Food and Drug Administration (FDA), whose apparent hostility to gays worried Curran. Because the "FDA has [a] long-standing aversion to gay blood donors," Curran claimed, "the extremes of panel recommendations could be: exclusion of any donor with indication of Hep. B; require screening to determine if donor is gay, then refuse donations." But, Curran insisted, an effective "messenger" who could "relate information to [the] gay community and media" might help block the panel from proposing or adopting such harsh policies.[38]

Attendees of the July 13 and 14 meetings sought to preemptively "confront the backlash leap to 'blame' AID[S] on gays" and "to negate patterns of association" within the larger discourse surrounding HIV/AIDS. Accordingly, they suggested alternatives to the draconian, antigay measures that were likely to be considered at the Expert Committee meeting. Since the "*MMWR* with information of hemophilia A/A.I.D.[S.] cases goes public on 7/16, [and] to NYTimes on 7/15 pm," the "Ad Hoc A.I.D.[S] Task Force" members hoped to "prepare an organized response to guide public opinion on issue of AID[S]/blood product relationship." They pressed for "donor-screening program[s]" that "exclude groupings (ie, not 'Are you gay?' but 'How many sexual contacts have you had in the last month?')," a position that anticipated the bans on "gay blood" that would be implemented in 1983 and beyond. For his part, Curran decried the fact that "screening for AID[S] is currently nonexistant [*sic*]" and that screening measures "under development are economically prohibitive on a large scale." As per Curran's recommendation, task force members also selected immunologist Dr. Roger Enlow and NGTF cofounder and biologist Bruce Voeller to serve on the Expert Committee. (After an illustrious career as a gay rights activist and biomedical researcher at the Rockefeller Institute, Voeller would die of AIDS-related causes in 1994.) These representatives would "make a strong statement for and from the gay community" and "challeng[e] heterosexual myths about homosexuality."[39]

The reactions of the ad hoc task force indicate that gay and lesbian activists and their allies recognized the power and privilege of people with hemophilia in the burgeoning national conversation on HIV/AIDS, several years before Ryan White became a household name. Curran himself lamented that "3 out of 22,000 hemophiliacs with AID[S] is considered a lot (epidemic)," perhaps underscoring the presumed disposability of other populations affected by the illness. Indeed, by the time the CDC published its *Morbidity and Mortality Weekly Report* concerning hemophilia and AIDS, hundreds of Americans—many of whom belonged to marginalized groups—had already succumbed to AIDS-related illnesses. Task force members acknowledged this apparent mismatch between the perceived value of people with hemophilia and that of MSM or intravenous drug users and hoped to "confront the probability of increased homophobia in reaction to [the] AID[S]/blood panic" or the idea that gays' "bad blood" now threatened less stigmatized populations.[40]

In this context, policymakers, lobbyists, and others pursued bans on blood donation by MSM. The Medical and Scientific Advisory Council of the NHF called for the exclusion of "high risk" blood and plasma donors in mid-January 1983, about six weeks before the US Public Health Service offered its first "cautiously worded, exclusionary recommendations" (in March 1983) concerning sexual behavior and blood donation.[41] The FDA was charged with overseeing "a largely voluntary effort to exclude as donors those who have the disease [HIV/AIDS] or its early symptoms and those in high-risk groups: sexually active homosexual or bisexual males, who have multiple partners; recent residents of Haiti; present or past abusers of intravenous drugs[;] and sexual partners of those in the high-risk category."[42] According to a March 1983 article published in the LGBTQ+ magazine *The Advocate*, the NHF was "the first major organization to urge the exclusion of gay donors," although its decision came on the heels of the Alpha Therapeutic Corporation's issuance of "a directive to its affiliate blood banks that all plasma donors be screened to exclude gay men and members of the other two high-risk groups."[43]

Roger Enlow and Bruce Voeller, who had been selected by the "Ad Hoc A.I.D.[S] Task Force" to serve as representatives on the Expert Committee, enjoyed some initial successes in their attempts to block bans against "gay blood."[44] But the NHF, the FDA, and other major players continued to discourage blood "donations from high-risk groups."[45] In 1986, the FDA "barred any man who had had sex with another man between 1977 and the present from donating blood." Only in the 2010s would these restrictions begin to loosen.[46] Yet these measures could not and did not prevent Ryan White and thousands of other people with hemophilia from contracting HIV.

Other, less exclusionary approaches might have yielded different results. As political scientist Patricia Siplon points out, a 1995 committee launched by Secretary of Health and Human Services Donna Shalala "found that the blood industry could have developed heat treatment processes before 1980, thereby preventing many of the AIDS cases among hemophiliacs that ultimately developed." The committee also determined that the FDA had coordinated too closely with "the blood banking and blood products complex," as Enlow and Voeller called it, which ultimately stymied attempts to screen, test, and treat blood products and thus to stop further transmission of HIV. The "profit motive," Siplon argues, dissuaded blood suppliers and pharmaceutical companies from recalling unscreened blood products, which would have cut into their bottom line. Such financial considerations delayed the transition from untreated to treated antihemophilic factor. Even in the mid-1980s, by which point the heat treatment of antihemophilic factor had become commonplace, the FDA refused "to require that manufacturers recall and destroy all untreated units." Only in 1989 would the FDA issue such a mandate.[47] The agency also rejected the NHF's demand for "the automatic recall of blood products associated with donors who were later diagnosed with AIDS."[48]

The NHF fared little better in the committee's report. Not unlike the FDA's enmeshment within "the blood banking and blood products complex," the NHF had become reliant on the for-profit blood and plasma industry. This "close and interdependent" relationship, committee members charged, spawned dubious NHF recommendations that "reflected conflicts of interest, were not adequately objective, and seriously compromised NHF's credibility."[49] Indeed, despite its endorsement of limited, targeted, "conservative" product recalls, the NHF and the Medical and Scientific Advisory Council routinely downplayed the risk to people with hemophilia and encouraged the continued use of concentrate as needed.[50] Experts such as the hematologist Oscar Ratnoff had long warned that blood-borne diseases could appear in pooled products such as Factor VIII. Since the mid-sixties—the dawn of the "golden era"—Ratnoff had vociferously supported the use of cryoprecipitate over concentrate. As the specter of AIDS loomed in the early 1980s, he urged those with hemophilia to "switch immediately," even though cryoprecipitate and fresh-frozen plasma were "less convenient" than concentrate, which could be administered at home. Perhaps unsurprisingly, Ratnoff encountered tremendous resistance among the NHF's medical advisors and the wider hemophilia community. "There is no conclusive evidence that cryoprecipitate or fresh frozen plasma will reduce the risk of AIDS," declared an NHF advisory released in December 1982.[51]

Considering the confidence with which the NHF advised people with hemophilia to "MAINTAIN THE USE OF CONCENTRATE" in the early 1980s—and the lack of urgency displayed by the FDA and the blood industry on the issue of HIV in the blood supply—thousands of people with hemophilia, including Ryan White, continued their Factor VIII regimens.[52] According to the CDC, about "half of the 16,000 hemophiliacs [in the United States] and over 12,000 recipients of blood transfusions became infected with HIV" from 1982 to 1984.[53] It is safe to assume that the overwhelming majority of those people died.

RYAN'S ROAD TO AIDS

Questions concerning disability and normality arose immediately after Ryan White's birth and subsequent hemophilia diagnosis. Basketball, of course, is king in Indiana, and Ryan was born during Bobby Knight's first year as head coach of the Indiana Hoosiers men's basketball team. (On the day that Ryan was born, Knight's Hoosiers beat the fourteenth-ranked Kansas Jayhawks at Assembly Hall in Bloomington.)[54] Before Ryan's hemophilia diagnosis, Jeanne—a Hoosier through and through—imagined that her newborn's stature and build (22.5 inches tall, just 7.8 pounds, "with big feet") would allow him to excel on the basketball court. "I looked at this long, thin baby and thought with joy, like a real Indiana sports fan: I got my basketball player!" When she learned that Ryan had hemophilia, she was dejected. "When they tell you that something is terribly wrong with your child," Jeanne wrote in 1997, "it takes a while to be able to think clearly about it." As Jeanne's and Ryan's public pronouncements indicate, "think[ing] clearly" about Ryan's interlocking maladies (first hemophilia and then AIDS) involved disavowing disability and striving for normality.[55]

In keeping with aspects of the "individual model of disability," which encourages disabled persons "to adapt to the[ir] environment through individual effort," the Whites often portrayed Ryan's hemophilia as largely attitudinal or psychological.[56] "I'd certainly rather not have hemophilia," Ryan admitted in his cowritten autobiography. "But if you feel sorry for yourself, you'll be so down you won't notice anything in life to enjoy." From an early age, Ryan explained, "I'd already decided that I didn't *have* hemophilia—I was living with it. You *can* feel well no matter what's wrong with you. I think that's the only way to think."[57] In that same vein, Jeanne claimed that she had avoided certain recommended precautions, such as placing a helmet on Ryan's head. These sorts of measures, according to Jeanne, would "teach [Ryan] to feel like he was sickly," and "handling this thing [hemophilia] was very much a matter of attitude." The Whites would take a similar tack following Ryan's AIDS diagnosis. In fact, Jeanne explicitly linked her son's spirited response to hemophilia with the courage he displayed in the face of AIDS. "I know that Ryan's positive attitude spilled over to help him when he had to deal with AIDS," she wrote.[58] This approach would help shape conceptions of Ryan's AIDS and establish the narrative frames employed in news media and pop cultural treatments of the White saga.

The view that Ryan's hemophilia (and later AIDS) could be "overcome" through positive thinking (and, later, education) conformed with contemporaneous cultural narratives that prized individual perseverance, rehabilitation, and productivity, particularly among adolescents. Such narratives—perhaps best exemplified by ABC's *After School Specials*, which "presented coming-of-age lessons through stories of the healthy overcoming of disability"—structured accounts of Ryan White's life.[59] For instance, in a short 1988 PBS documentary about Ryan White, which was subsequently nominated for an Emmy Award, a Brooklyn fifth-grader asks Ryan, "What's it like to be a hemophiliac?" In his response, Ryan notes that he refuses to let hemophilia constrict his movements. Although doctors advised him not to ride a bike, he always had, he tells a classroom full of fifth-graders. "I just try to do everything like everybody else—always have, always will." The rest of the documentary echoes Ryan's claims, particularly those pertaining to hemophilia and "normality." As scenes of Ryan delivering newspapers on his bicycle appear onscreen—images that connote "normal" boyhood—the documentary's narrator details how AIDS upended the boy's life. "Until 1984," the year of his AIDS diagnosis, "Ryan White lived like any other kid in Kokomo, Indiana—riding his bike, going to school, and playing with his dog Barney." The documentary thus replicates the Whites' conception of Ryan's hemophilia as a minor inconvenience, one that a resilient individual could conceivably overcome.[60]

Likewise, Ryan and his mother sought to distinguish the young boy from more severely impaired or less "fortunate" individuals, a maneuver that intersected with broader efforts to situate Ryan atop "a hierarchy of victimhood" within the "moral epidemic" of AIDS.[61] "Hemophilia isn't the worst problem a kid can have," Ryan indicated in his coauthored autobiography. During stints at the hospital, he "met plenty of kids in bigger trouble than [he] was"—those battling cancer, those with "horrible burns," those with mental or intellectual disabilities, and those with "all kinds of defects and other diseases" that required "operation after operation."[62] "I'm just glad all that's wrong with me is my hemophilia," Ryan reportedly told his mother. Jeanne counted her blessings following Ryan's hemophilia diagnosis. "Look at all the people who can't have kids at all, I said to myself. Think how much luckier you are than they," she exclaimed in her autobiography. "I kept remembering one of Grandma Helen's sayings, 'I wept that I had no shoes, until I met a man who had no feet.'"[63] The use of this aphorism suggests that Jeanne and her grandmother both equated physical impairment with misfortune and took pains to distance Ryan from populations deserving of pity.

If "hemophilia didn't seem that bad," in Ryan's words, it was largely due to the advent and growing accessibility of Factor VIII. By the time Ryan turned five, his doctors had authorized him to receive Factor VIII injections at home. Although Jeanne insisted that she was "not smart enough to give shots," she learned "how to tie a tourniquet around [Ryan's] arm, find a vein," and administer the injections safely and effectively. Ryan received these injections some "two or three times a week," sometimes more frequently whenever he sustained a bleed. Factor VIII thus became a fundamental part of life in the White household. Ryan even "took to calling it 'Old Faithful' because it worked so well," while Jeanne celebrated the fact that her "innocent little boy" had been "born in the era of Factor VIII."[64]

Jeanne's father, Thomas Hale, viewed Factor VIII with suspicion, however. "He had heard a rumor, from someone at Riley [Hospital for Children in Indianapolis] or someone at the pharmacy," Jeanne recounted, "that the more you took the Factor, the more likely you were to develop an inhibitor reaction which would make it less and less effective as time went by."[65] And as AIDS began to appear in older individuals with hemophilia, Hale implored his daughter to stop treating Ryan with Factor. "Jeanne, I'm just scared to death Ryan's going to catch AIDS," he explained. Ryan apparently sought to alleviate his grandfather's fears by recalling an article in *Time* magazine, which revealed "that less than one percent of hemophiliacs have AIDS, and they're older guys—not kids." Ryan speculated, "Maybe they're gay too, and got AIDS that way."[66]

But Thomas Hale's fears proved well-founded. His grandson started to feel chronically ill in the summer of 1984, not long after the Whites had moved from Windfall, Indiana, following Jeanne's second divorce, to nearby Kokomo, Jeanne's hometown. (Jeanne and Wayne White, Ryan's father, had divorced when Ryan was seven, and her marriage to Steve Ford ended in 1982.)[67] Ryan was twelve and a half at the time and "looking forward to turning into a typical obnoxious teenager." But constant night sweats, diarrhea, lethargy, and stomach cramps put a damper on his transition from childhood to adolescence. By the time Ryan turned thirteen on December 6, 1984, he had reached a breaking point. "Mom, you've got to do something," he pleaded. "I can't even get off the school bus without being tired. I can't figure out what's wrong." After Ryan ran a fever of 104 degrees the following weekend, Jeanne took him to the hospital in Kokomo, where an X-ray revealed that he had pneumonia in both lungs. Antibiotics failed to treat the pneumonia, so Ryan was transferred to Riley Hospital for Children in Indianapolis. There, Jeanne and Ryan met with Dr. Martin Kleiman, an expert in pediatric infectious diseases. Given Ryan's severe hemophilia and reliance on Factor VIII, Kleiman suspected that his pneumonia was viral rather than bacterial, hence the inefficacy of the antibiotic regimen. Specifically, Kleiman believed Pneumocystis carinii pneumonia to be the culprit.[68]

PCP usually poses few problems, but it can be devastating for immunocompromised individuals. Alongside Kaposi's sarcoma, PCP served as one of the rare opportunistic infections that alerted clinicians to the existence of a new disease in the early 1980s.[69] A Kaposi's sarcoma or PCP diagnosis often worked as a de facto AIDS diagnosis, particularly before the introduction of reliable HIV antibody testing in the mid- to late eighties. Thus, when a biopsy conducted on Ryan White's lungs came back positive for PCP, it essentially confirmed that he had AIDS. Though it was unclear precisely when Ryan had contracted HIV, which subsequently led to AIDS, Kleiman speculated that Ryan might have been infected as early as 1982 or 1983, well before the widespread use of heat treatment to eliminate HIV, hepatitis, and other viruses from the blood supply. Jeanne initially hid the diagnosis from her son, but this position became increasingly untenable as the news spread around the hospital and beyond. With Christmas fast approaching, Jeanne vowed to tell Ryan on Boxing Day, after he had received his new computer and other gifts.[70]

A burglary at the Whites' residence further spoiled the family's Christmas and also exposed some of the fault lines along which the Ryan White story would unfold in the coming years. The culprits had broken in through the back door of the Whites' house and made off with the computer Jeanne had purchased for Ryan as well as the VCR she had planned to gift her daughter, Andrea. According to Ryan's coauthored autobiography, "The robbers knew I was in the hospital with AIDS. Word was racing around our neighborhood and our Methodist church in Kokomo."[71] This claim underscored the supposed cruelty of a broad swath of Kokomo's population, a theme that would structure the dominant news media and pop culture narratives around the Ryan White saga. However, the Christmas Eve burglary was just one of several "B&Es and thefts" reported to the Howard County sheriff's office between mid-November 1984 and January 1, 1985. Various locals, the sheriff's department, and historian Allen Safianow also insisted that the alleged burglars had no knowledge of the boy's AIDS diagnosis. Indeed, while news of Ryan's illness likely spread around town in the weeks following his diagnosis, the Whites did not go public with the news until early March 1985. In oral history interviews conducted in the twenty-first century, furthermore, several locals suggested that the Whites' memoirs and the 1989 made-for-television film *The Ryan White Story* concealed the Kokomo community's generous response to the Christmastime burglary. "What about the people

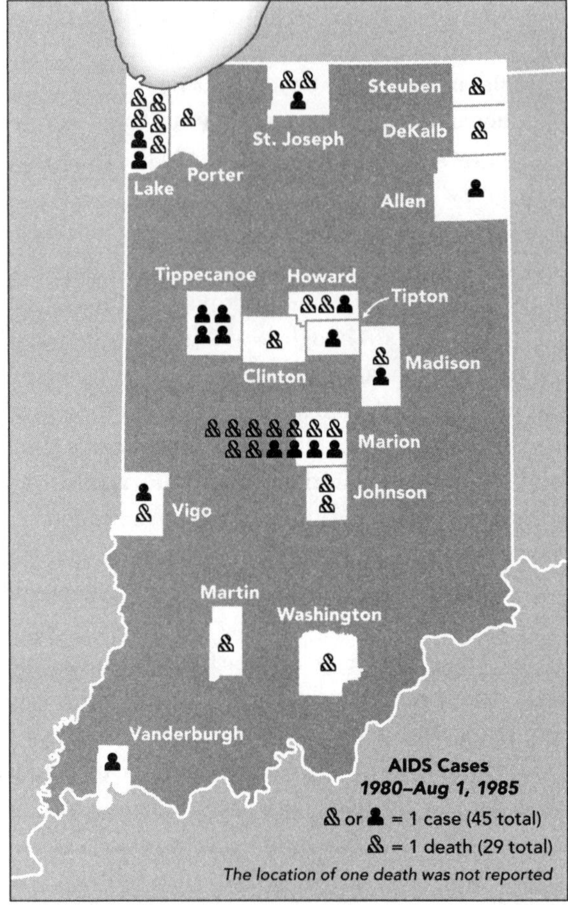

Distribution of known AIDS cases in Indiana counties from 1980 to August 1, 1985. Map by Daniel Huffman and based on a map featured in Carol Elrod, "AIDS: Now a Household Word, It's Invading 'Straight' World," *Indianapolis Star*, August 4, 1985, 1A, 20A.

in the community that replaced those Christmas presents?" asked Wanda Bilodeau, the sister of Ryan's best friend, Heath Bowen.[72]

Ryan's cowritten autobiography also blamed the burglary on the Whites' "druggy neighbors," one of many subtle maneuvers taken by the Whites and their supporters to distinguish Ryan from more "deviant" or marginalized populations—including those addicted to drugs, severely disabled people, and gay people. Elsewhere in the autobiography, for example, Ryan and his coauthor, Ann Marie Cunningham, detailed the various populations most susceptible to HIV infection: gay men, intravenous drug users, and people with hemophilia. While they attached no value judgments to gay men or people with hemophilia, they marshaled Ryan's medical history to stigmatize those who use drugs, intravenous or not. "After all the times I've been stuck and all the medicine I've had to take," Ryan wrote with the help of his coauthor, "I can't imagine anyone actually *wanting* to use needles or drugs. But people do. They should find out what it's like to *have* to take drugs *all* the time."[73] Not only did this passage fundamentally misapprehend the nature of drug use and addiction; it also fortified the "hierarchy of victimhood" that decisively shaped coverage and understandings of HIV/AIDS, particularly in the 1980s and 1990s. This rhetorical move also deserves to be considered alongside Ryan's efforts to differentiate himself from more severely disabled young people.

In that vein, when Jeanne informed Ryan that he was now living with AIDS, he responded by likening the illness to his hemophilia and holding fast to his vision of "normality." Upon learning of his diagnosis, he "thought a minute" and asked himself, "So what was the big deal about AIDS? I was a hemophiliac," Ryan reasoned, "so I already had my limits. But I'd been having an okay time, anyway. I certainly wasn't about to die yet. Why not just get back to being a normal kid?" Ryan then told his mother, "Let's just pretend I don't have it." He elaborated, "I just don't want everybody feeling sorry for me and thinking 'Poor little Ryan, he's dying.' I just want to make believe I don't have AIDS and do what I want to do."[74] Just as Ryan and, at times, his mother had downplayed the severity of his hemophilia and touted the power of positive thinking in dealing with the illness, they approached AIDS as a similar obstacle that could be overcome, or at least managed, through positivity and resilience. This perspective—which Ryan's allies in the news media and entertainment industries would promote and celebrate—helped inform Ryan's quest for "normality," which in turn would propel his efforts to return to school in the Kokomo area.

NEVER NORMAL?

Ryan had contracted a "gay disease" that had supposedly spread from a marginalized population to a misunderstood yet unstigmatized group that had long sought to appear "normal."[75] Even Jeanne White, in an attempt to diminish antigay stigma several months after Ryan's diagnosis, reinforced the notion that the illness her son now carried had originated in, or had been spread primarily by, gay men. "When they told me" about the results of Ryan's biopsy, "I got mad," Jeanne told the *Kokomo Tribune* in March 1985. "I wasn't mad at them. I wasn't mad at the gays. I was mad because I couldn't believe that the factor that he had been taking all his life to keep him alive was the very thing that was killing him now." In that same *Tribune* article, Jeanne conveyed her excitement about that upcoming summer, during which, she assumed, the Whites could "do some things as a family before [Ryan] has to get back to school."[76] Little did Jeanne know that officials at the Western School Corporation would bar Ryan from attending Western Middle School, all while promising to provide him with "an education outside of the normal school setting."[77] And little did she know that an ensuing legal battle would transform her son into a curious kind of celebrity.

Ryan's story resonated with the news media and the broader public for a variety of reasons, but chief among them was his "exceptional" status in the world of AIDS, a status attributable in large part to his hemophilia. Because Ryan had acquired HIV through contaminated blood products—that is, "through no fault of his own," as many observers imagined it—he was, in the words of one *Indianapolis Star* reader, an "innocent victim of a terrible disease that spread to the 'straight' population from the homosexual community."[78] The boy's desire to "get back to being a normal kid" also resonated widely, because Ryan White was legible as a "normal" child, in spite of his hemophilia and AIDS.[79] In other words, his whiteness, youth, middle-class status, and boyish charisma and charm made him relatable, while his heterosexuality, sickness, and slight stature (a product of his AIDS) accentuated his youth and rendered him vulnerable and nonthreatening, unlike so many other PWAs. Ryan's thirst for "normality," articulated and validated through a sympathetic national news media apparatus, also served as a subtle refutation of disability and "deviance." As Ryan embarked on a prolonged struggle to return to Western Middle School in person, he would become a household name and a "quiet hero" in ways that few other PWAs or disabled people could imagine.[80]

CHAPTER TWO

NORMAL ACTIVITIES

In this culture, how we think about disease determines who lives and who dies. . . . The power to define disease and normality makes AIDS a political issue.

Evelynn Hammonds, "Race, Sex, AIDS: The Construction of 'Other,'" 1987

Ryan White just wanted to go back to school. In much the same way that he had handled hemophilia, Ryan vowed not to let his AIDS diagnosis spoil his otherwise "normal" childhood. A key component of living like a "normal kid," Ryan's deeply held wish, was attending school and socializing with friends and acquaintances.[1] Although he was too sick to return to Western Middle School (WMS) for the remainder of the 1984–85 academic year, he planned on coming back in the fall of 1985. WMS officials seemed open to the idea, at least in public. A March 1985 *Kokomo Tribune* article in which the Whites publicly disclosed Ryan's diagnosis indicated that officials were "considering . . . perhaps permitting [Ryan] to return to school at the beginning of next school year."[2] Yet on July 30, 1985, Western School Corporation (WSC) superintendent J. O. Smith blocked Ryan from attending WMS because he was living with AIDS.[3] Smith's decision prompted the White family to file a lawsuit in US district court a week later, setting the stage for a legal battle that would last for most of the 1985–86 academic year.

These developments not only ignited a media firestorm, as outlets from *NBC Nightly News* to the *Chicago Tribune* to ABC's *Nightline* picked up the story, but also divided locals and outsiders alike into competing camps, with some vociferously opposing Ryan's campaign to return to school and others strongly supporting it.[4] In the service of their respective causes, these competing camps relied on different conceptions of normality, innocence, risk, and education. For those in Kokomo and beyond who backed Ryan's bid to return to Western, Ryan was a "regular kid" who deserved conventional in-person schooling.[5] His need for a "normal education," as one supporter later put it, aligned with the imperative to properly educate the public about the causes of HIV/AIDS.[6] For his opponents, Ryan was too ill and frail to attend school, and his disease posed a threat to the health and safety of his classmates and teachers, as well as others who lived in Kokomo, Russiaville, and surrounding towns. To justify their campaign to keep Ryan out of Western Middle School, many pointed to lingering questions about AIDS, even among some medical professionals, while insisting that they knew more about the disease than the average person on the street.[7]

Ultimately Ryan and his allies won out, and Ryan returned to school at Western in 1986. This victory not only cemented Ryan's status as a celebrity, an AIDS ambassador, and an exceptional yet normal victim but also revealed a broader cultural and political emphasis on education, "awareness," and personal responsibility in the AIDS epidemic. Both developments served to individualize HIV/AIDS and foreclose opportunities for more collective, structural responses to the crisis.

SCHOOL'S OUT

On the surface, Ryan seemed like just another seventh grader at Western Middle School. He was new to WMS in the fall of 1984, having moved to Kokomo earlier that year from Windfall, Indiana, about eighteen miles away. While living in Windfall, Ryan attended Tri-Central Junior High in nearby Sharpsville, where he earned mostly As and Bs (and a couple of Cs). He received similar grades (plus one D) in his first semester at Western Middle School.[8] As WMS principal Ron Colby put it, "Ryan was functioning at an average to above average level the 1st and 2nd 6 weeks [*sic*] grading period at Western Middle School the fall semester of 1984–85," just before his hospitalization and subsequent AIDS diagnosis in December 1984. The boy also exhibited no "abnormal emotional behavior" and "appeared to socialize with his peers in a normal fashion for a 7th grader new to the school system."[9] Though Ryan had severe hemophilia, Jeanne White had advised Colby and school nurse Bev Ashcraft on her son's condition. Despite the potential dangers that a child with hemophilia might face in a middle school setting—namely horseplay and other activities that could cause internal bleeding—Colby, Ashcraft, and other WMS officials seemed confident in their ability to care for Ryan. According to Colby, there had been some "concern when school first started in '84," but Ryan's severe hemophilia ultimately presented "no major problem[s] until Nov[ember]—when we could

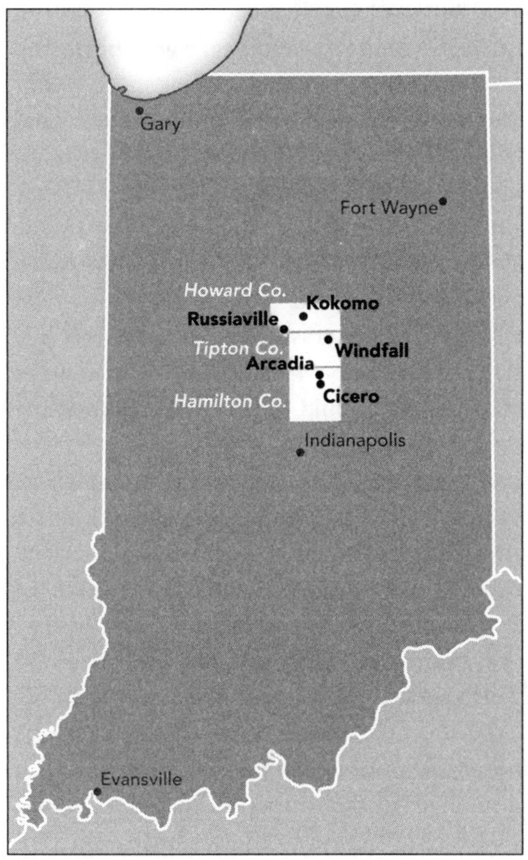

Key sites in the Ryan White story. Map by Daniel Huffman.

not stop [a] nosebleed."[10] Ryan ultimately survived that incident, just as he survived so many other health scares.

Yet even though Ryan intended to approach AIDS as he had approached hemophilia, AIDS was a different beast entirely for school officials and other locals. Accordingly, Ryan's AIDS prompted a different set of responses from teachers, administrators, and others in the Kokomo area, especially as the fall 1985 semester drew nearer. By then, the medical community had confirmed that HIV spread mainly through particular sexual activities, needle-sharing, blood products, and blood transfusions—and not through casual contact. Nevertheless, many area parents and school administrators sought clarity on the specific issue of students with AIDS in schools. In the run-up to the 1985–86 academic year, WSC and WMS teachers and administrators awaited guidance from local, state, or federal health officials on the matter.

The Indiana State Board of Health (ISBH) supplied such guidance only in late July 1985, less than a month before the new school year was to begin and just days before students were to formally enroll at WMS.[11]

Released on July 30, 1985, the ISBH report—spurred by Ryan's case and based on similar guidelines developed in Connecticut and Florida—strongly affirmed the right of children with AIDS to attend school.[12] "No evidence exists to support transmission of the disease by casual contact or by the airborne route," the ISBH guidelines read. "All evidence regarding the transmission of AIDS indicates that the type of contact between persons which normally occurs in a school setting should not result in the transmission of the AIDS virus."[13] That same day, possibly before he had the state guidelines in hand, J. O. Smith announced that Ryan would be barred from attending WMS in person.

Smith and his supporters justified the decision in several interlocking ways. First and foremost, they pointed to lingering questions about HIV's potential modes of transmission. Next, they argued that Ryan's physical attendance could threaten the health and well-being of everyone in the school (including Ryan himself) and in the surrounding community. Finally, they contended that the onerous safeguards recommended by the ISBH would be difficult to implement and also spoke to the potential communicability of HIV.

Smith cited "unknowns and uncertainties [about AIDS]" as a reason to keep Ryan out of school, and he insisted that the ISBH guidelines raised more questions than they answered.[14] "There's the misconception that there's only one way to catch AIDS[:] through sexual intercourse," Smith told the *Kokomo Tribune* shortly after the ISBH released its recommendations. "But the guidelines we've received indicate that the exchange of certain other body fluids could present a danger to other students."[15] As Smith put it on the *CBS Evening News* on July 31, "What we know about it, combined with what we don't know, just makes it too big a problem and too many question marks."[16] Western School Board president Dan Carter sounded similar notes in an interview with the *Tribune*. "As long as we have any question that might affect the health of any student, we have to take a safe route" by keeping Ryan out of school.[17]

WSC officials certainly had plenty of questions. A week after the release of the state guidelines, WSC representatives submitted an extensive list of queries to the ISBH. Their exacting questions sowed confusion about the communicability of HIV/AIDS and thus cast doubt on the validity of the ISBH's claims. "Is AIDS a communicable disease?" the authors of the WSC memo asked. "Is AIDS transmittable by saliva? coughing? sneezing? perspiration?" While the ISBH guidelines had specified that HIV could not be transmitted through "casual contact," WSC officials wondered, "What constitutes 'casual contact'?" and "Is there a difference between 'casual contact' at home and at school?"[18] That the ISBH identified certain precautions to be taken in the event of a "spill" involving the bodily fluids of a child with AIDS raised red flags. Some observers interpreted this as proof of HIV's extreme transmissibility. Smith also suggested that these recommended safeguards—namely the use of "gloves, bleach, and leakproof bags"—were burdensome, presumably because the school corporation was rural, fairly small, and in financial straits.[19] In Smith's words, Ryan's physical presence at WMS would be "a situation we are not prepared to cope with."[20]

The decision to deny entry to Ryan might have remained a relatively minor local controversy had it not come down just as the world learned of actor Rock Hudson's bout with AIDS. Though Hudson had been diagnosed in 1984, news of his illness broke only in late July 1985. Hudson thus became, as the *Indianapolis Star* put it, "the first person with international recognition to announce he has the disease."[21] Hudson's fame made his illness noteworthy and shocking, but so too did his status as a heterosexual icon. Hudson had long personified normative masculinity on the big screen, especially during Hollywood's "golden age"—starring alongside Elizabeth Taylor in the epic *Giant* (1956) and Doris Day in several popular romantic comedies, including *Pillow Talk* (1959). Accordingly, news of Hudson's diagnosis heightened public interest in the AIDS epidemic and stoked fears about the disease's movement beyond the established "risk groups" (the so-called four Hs: homosexuals, hemophiliacs, heroin users, and Haitians).[22] Just days after Smith's decision, the *Indianapolis Star* ran a front-page article (next to a story about Ryan White) spotlighting the public's growing concerns about AIDS. "Now a Household Word," the headline read, "It's Invading 'Straight' World."[23]

Smith's decision brought national and international attention to Kokomo, Russiaville, and the small communities surrounding them. And because AIDS was "now a household word," Ryan White soon became a household name, a widely celebrated figure with a small army backing his bid to return to school. "It all broke loose," Dan Carter explained in a 2011 oral history interview. "Then the whole country starts swooping down on us [saying], 'How dare you?'"[24] Given how quiet this part of north-central Indiana was (and is), it is easy to understand why locals might have been overwhelmed by the national and international news media coverage. Just two days after

Smith's decision, the front page of the *Kokomo Tribune* included a short article called "Case in the Spotlight," which began, "The case of Ryan White has gained attention nationwide through the news media."[25] The story—surrounded by three others related to the Ryan White saga—revealed just how unprecedented these developments were for people in the Kokomo area.

With this publicity came scrutiny and criticism, as Carter suggested, and also tremendous sympathy for Ryan. At a moment in which AIDS seemed to be on everyone's mind, Ryan emerged as a nearly unassailable figure without the presumed baggage of other people with AIDS. In the wake of Smith's decision, Ryan received encouraging letters and other forms of support from people around the world. By contrast, many of the letters sent to Smith and WMS principal Ron Colby in 1985 and beyond expressed admiration for White and disdain for school administrators and the residents of the Kokomo area, more generally. Ryan White's supporters often emphasized "innocence" and the concept of "normality" in their appeals, with some clearly motivated by pity for the young person with hemophilia—and now AIDS.

After reading about Ryan in the summer of 1985, Susan O'Brien—who hailed from the affluent Chicago suburb of Wayne—informed J. O. Smith that she was "heartsick over what you've done to this boy." O'Brien observed that Ryan had contracted HIV "through no fault of his own," apparently unlike the men who had sex with men or the injecting drug users who had been infected by participating in risky, illicit activities. Despite Ryan's innocence, O'Brien wrote, Smith had "cruelly exclude[d] him from his right to school and a normal life." O'Brien moved seamlessly between innocence, normality, and school attendance in her analysis of Ryan's ordeal, while the deviants presumably at fault for their infections warranted little sympathy or consideration.[26] Jane Tan, a fifteen-year-old Chinese girl living in the Philippines, seemed to agree, as she linked normal boyhood to "health" and freedom from "that disease." "You don't deserve to have that disease," she told Ryan in a September 1985 letter. "You deserve to be just like any other healthy boys [*sic*]."[27] For Irene Holleran of Rochester, New York, Smith's decision was "abhorable [*sic*]," especially considering the "physical and emotional pain" and "lack of a normal childhood and social life" to which Ryan had already been subjected due to his severe hemophilia. "What next! Where is your humanitarianism!" Holleran asked, thus imploring Smith to take pity on Ryan by giving him a taste of normality.[28]

Ryan's supporters also advanced a narrow vision of education that would structure Ryan White's very public life from 1985 until his death in 1990.

These understandings of education and AIDS awareness focused not on safer-sex practices or on the inequities that made some groups more susceptible to infection, illness, and death—what some scholars call the social determinants of health. Rather, calls for greater awareness concentrated on the ways in which HIV could and could not be transmitted—an approach that reinforced the stigmas associated with anal sex and intravenous drug use, widened the perceived gap between supposedly innocent and guilty people with AIDS, and suggested that HIV/AIDS did not represent a threat to most people outside of particular "risk groups."[29] Such understandings of education also served to endow Ryan's campaign to return to school with significant meaning. Not only was Ryan White fighting for his own education; he was fighting to educate the broader public about AIDS.

Writing to Western School Corporation superintendent J. O. Smith in August 1985, Ina Sherman—the mother of a young woman who would die of AIDS-related causes the following year—declared that her letter "concerns all people, especially those of you purporting to be educators." Because of her daughter's illness, Sherman wrote, "all of our family have dedicated themselves to *education*! Perhaps, since this should be your primary goal, I can help you to be true educators and to achieve that goal." In an effort to educate Smith and his colleagues, Sherman shared excerpts from an August 1985 *Washington Post* article, which stressed that HIV "does not appear to be spread through casual contact, but rather through [the] intimate exchange of body fluids." Sherman explained that she worked mightily to combat the sort of "fear and ignorance" that supposedly animated Smith's decision. "There is no reason to deny this boy an education—in school—so long as his energy and health permit him to attend classes." Again underscoring the importance of education, Sherman ended her letter with a plea to "let us help you and people like Ryan White!" She urged Smith not to "deny this boy an education—in school—and the closeness of his peers and friends."[30] In her letter, Susan O'Brien similarly implored Smith: "You must educate the people in your town," she wrote. "All studies show that AIDS is transmitted by intense sexual contact (or blood transfusions). . . . I implore you to change your decision based on incorrect information, fear, and politics."[31]

Just as Ryan White's supporters foregrounded his youth, normality, and right to an education in their appeals, those who sought to keep Ryan out of WMS recognized his near unassailability as an innocent and sickly child. Accordingly, Ryan's detractors rarely impugned his character in public. In fact, many played up concerns about the teenager's well-being. At the same time, they privileged the health and safety of other people (particularly children) supposedly threatened by Ryan's illness. In the days after Smith barred Ryan White from WSC schools, a visible and vocal group of Kokomo-area residents and parents showed their support for Smith's decision. Describing herself as a "concerned parent," Mitzie Johnson and her husband, David, circulated a petition backing Smith's ruling. According to the *Kokomo Tribune*, the petition received "near-unanimous support" from the Johnsons' neighbors. Tellingly, the petition offered "prayers . . . to Ryan and his family" while also noting that the undersigned "must back Mr. Smith's decision until more evidence is gathered to guarantee the safety of our children as well as Ryan's."[32]

A week later, Mitzie Johnson organized a meeting of what the *Tribune* called "worried parents," most of whom opposed Ryan's bid to attend school at WMS. Over 300 people attended the meeting held in Western High School's cafeteria—including Paula Adair, president of the Western Teachers Association, which supported Smith's decision. "As teachers, we are concerned about Ryan," Adair told the crowd gathered at Western High School. "We are concerned about every student. . . . We're also concerned about the response other students will have to Ryan. Teachers are responsible for the social and educational well being of the student. Peer pressure will be a big factor. It can't be assumed that children will not have fears."[33] Though perhaps cynical, Adair's acknowledgment that Ryan could be bullied or mistreated at school underscored Ryan's perceived innocence and vulnerability. Mitzie Johnson offered additional support for Ryan during the meeting. "Not that I don't feel for Ryan. I do. But his disease is fatal," Johnson declared, gesturing not only to the threat that Ryan White ostensibly presented to her child and others, but also to Ryan's presumed frailty and proximity to death.[34] Johnson would soon spearhead an organization called Concerned Citizens and Parents of Children Attending Western School Corporation, which provided vital support for the WSC in its courtroom battles against Ryan and his family.

By September 1985, the inclusion of HIV-positive students and students with AIDS in the classroom had become a contentious national issue. Ryan White's youth, innocence, and compelling pursuit of normality indirectly forced President Ronald Reagan to address the AIDS crisis for the first time. Shortly after White and his family began waging their battle against the Western School Corporation, reporters at a September 17 press conference urged Reagan to discuss the controversy over students with AIDS. He did, although he refused to affirm the right of children with HIV/AIDS to attend school. When asked to imagine that he had younger children and to indicate whether he would "send them to a school with a child who had AIDS," Reagan equivocated. "I can well understand the plight of the parents," the president asserted. "I also have compassion," he continued, "for the child that has this [AIDS] and doesn't know . . . why somehow he is now an outcast and can no longer associate with his playmates and schoolmates."[35] Reagan's comments disappointed health officials like Paul Volberding, an oncologist and the director of the AIDS clinic at San Francisco General Hospital. "I don't think the President's remarks reflect what most experts in the field feel about that issue," Volberding observed. "Most of us feel that kids with AIDS should be allowed to participate in normal activities."[36] With little federal leadership on AIDS, debates about children with HIV/AIDS in schools would continue to rage in the courtroom, the press, and the interpersonal sphere, from Connecticut to the Bronx to Florida, where locals tormented and eventually banished the Ray brothers, who also had hemophilia. But the Ryan White case would loom largest.

FROM THE CLASSROOM TO THE COURTROOM

Jeanne White was not a litigious person.[37] But as the White family attorney, Charles R. Vaughan Sr., explained in the days following Smith's ruling, Ryan was "entitled under civil rights to be in the environment of other students." The WSC's vow to provide Ryan with a private tutor or a telephone hookup to his classroom was "unacceptable," declared Vaughan. And so, a little over a week after Smith blocked Ryan from in-person classes, Vaughan filed a lawsuit on behalf of the Whites against the WSC in US district court in Indianapolis.[38] As Vaughan's remarks suggested, the Whites' legal action turned on the idea that Ryan was a normal boy who deserved to learn alongside other normal children.

The Whites' legal saga got off to a rocky start, however. The US district court judge assigned to the case ruled that Vaughan and the Whites must "follow proper administrative procedure" within the school system before turning to the courts.[39] They did just that, meeting with school officials in a process that attorney Vaughan considered not only futile but also onerous and cruel—given that, according to some estimates, Ryan might live for only another year or two. "We're going to have a case conference and they're going to find against us," he told the *Kokomo Tribune* in mid-September. As Vaughan saw it, the case conference, scheduled for September 19, was "the first step in a long line of exhausting administrative remedies we must do. We'll meet with the designated officers of the school corporation, the principal, maybe the superintendent. They'll forward a report to the superintendent. He can change, modify, or adopt their recommendation. We can appeal that."[40] After the case had traveled through the appropriate administrative channels at the local level, it would be reviewed by Indiana's Department of Education and then its Board of Special Education Appeals. "Only after all of those proceedings were concluded," historian and lawyer Ruth Reichard writes, "would the federal district court assume jurisdiction" on Ryan's case, a process that would take several months.[41] "Ryan's doctors say he has only two years to live," NBC's Mary Nissenson had reported on the *Nightly News* the previous month, "so several months seem like a very long time to him." "My greatest fear," Vaughan noted during the same *Nightly News* story, "is that Ryan will never get educated in the classroom. That's my greatest fear. That's a right I think he has."[42]

Though Vaughan expected WSC officials to stand firm in their decision to bar Ryan from attending classes in person, these initial administrative steps enabled Vaughan and the Whites to refine and further publicize their arguments in support of Ryan's campaign. In administrative meetings and news media interviews, Ryan and his representatives portrayed the young boy as normal while often pointing to his interlocking disabilities of hemophilia and AIDS. With these rhetorical moves, Ryan and his supporters could have it both ways: Ryan could be a normal boy who deserved a normal education *and* a gravely ill, pitiable child who deserved to spend his final days, weeks, months, or years with his friends and teachers. At least initially, Vaughan defended Ryan's right to return to school by citing the federal Rehabilitation Act of 1973 and the federal Education for All Handicapped Children Act of 1975, both of which focused on the needs of children with disabilities.[43] At the same time, because he believed that Ryan could "function in normal school," according to handwritten notes taken during the aforementioned September 19 case conference, Vaughan hoped that Ryan could be "mainstreamed."[44] As WMS principal Ron Colby put it, "Vaughan questioned any impairment of alertness or inability to function in a regular school program." Ryan also "want[ed] social activities," Vaughan told those gathered at the case conference and claimed that Ryan's "health problems may be because he is home." Vaughan thus highlighted the supposed psychological and attitudinal dimensions of Ryan's overlapping disabilities. The boy's health would improve, Vaughan implied, if he could simply return to Western Middle School.[45]

Just as Vaughan feared, this case conference changed nothing, as conference chairman Ron Colby "recommended continued home instruction for

Ryan" and Smith reinforced his initial ruling keeping Ryan out of school. It "was the most predictable decision in the world," Vaughan stated, and it further signaled the WSC's willingness to curtail Ryan's civil rights, which "caused him severe trauma." As Vaughan argued in the *Tribune* just after the decision in early October, "From a psychological view, Ryan's spirit has gone downhill since [WSC superintendent J. O.] Smith told him he can't go to school. That's a denial of his civil rights to obtain an education in a classroom." The "continued denial to let Ryan in is also continuing to do him harm, physically and emotionally," Vaughan insisted.[46]

Following the October 1985 ruling, Vaughan also publicly derided Smith for his presumed "lack of knowledge" concerning AIDS. "All medical evidence overwhelmingly substantiates AIDS can't be contracted through casual classroom contact," he declared. For Vaughan, school officials were "reacting emotionally rather than to medical evidence." Here, Vaughan portrayed his opponents as willfully ignorant and underlined the importance of "education," broadly conceived, in Ryan's case.[47]

But contrary to Vaughan's claims—which prefigured a national narrative concerning the presumed backwardness and closed-mindedness of Kokomo and Russiaville residents—WSC officials and ordinary locals accepted most features of the scientific consensus regarding AIDS. Notably, they seemed to recognize the low risk of transmitting HIV in a classroom or school setting. They nonetheless bristled at the idea of exposing HIV-negative students to such a risk, and they emphasized the protean and contested nature of medical knowledge about HIV/AIDS. "The risk of spreading the AIDS disease, however small, as far as we know today, is still a risk and the consequences are catastrophic," Ron Colby wrote in his opinion following the September 19 case conference. Colby explained that he "[did] not believe in *absolute guarantees* with any diseases know [*sic*] to man today," yet he called for more research on AIDS "before Western requires students to come into even casual contact with a person known to suffer from this illness."[48] Some concerned parents *did* demand such a guarantee (that children would not contract HIV if Ryan were to attend WMS in person). However, most of Ryan's opponents in the Kokomo area seemed to acknowledge that HIV transmission was highly unlikely, but not impossible, outside of certain activities. "The CDC says it is very difficult to catch AIDS," Mitzie Johnson announced to parents gathered at the WMS gymnasium in late September. "Maybe so. But I don't think AIDS is as difficult to catch as they'd like to lead us to believe."[49] These doubts, however slight, helped block Ryan's path to Western Middle School in the fall of 1985.

They weren't the only obstacles in Ryan's way. The young Hoosier was also struggling with a respiratory illness that kept him in the hospital for much of the fall.[50] Worse still, perhaps, when Ryan was healthy enough to learn, he had to do so via a phone hookup in his bedroom, a far cry from the "normal school" experience for which he and his supporters were petitioning.[51] While the local and national press expressed interest in the "special telephone line linking [Ryan's] home to his seventh-grade classroom"—a sign of the techno-optimism that defined the late twentieth century—the technology simply wasn't up to snuff. Reporting on the phone hookup in August 1985, United Press International lamented, "The sound quality for the first day of school was good at the school, but poor in Ryan's bedroom, which he uses as a classroom."[52] Ryan hated it. "It stinks!" he chuckled in a clip broadcast on *NBC Nightly News* and ABC's *World News Tonight*. "You can't hear anything." His sunny disposition giving way to disappointment, he then solemnly stated, "It's all muffled."[53] As ABC's Jerry King put it, "It was a frustrating day for Ryan White."[54]

Ryan's frustration, and the technical difficulties that caused it, spurred teleconferencing organizations and vendors to take action. "We saw the problems Ryan was having with the audio and we figured we could improve on that," one representative from the telecommunications company Westell remarked. "A story this big was giving such a bad name to teleconferencing that we thought this was a chance to get some good publicity for us and for teleconferencing in general."[55] With the help of such private vendors, Ryan's connection had improved by mid- to late September, but the remote hookup still couldn't compare to the experience of in-person education.[56] When the *Kokomo Tribune* covered Ryan's return to remote schooling in November 1985 after his forty-four-day stint in the hospital, its headline read, "Back to 'School.'" The paper therefore implied that White's "homebound" education was inferior to, or at least wholly different from, learning "in a normal school setting," as Ron Colby called it.[57] By portraying in-person education as normative and therefore desirable, the *Tribune* seemed to express support for White's campaign to return to Western Middle School.[58]

Debates over medical knowledge, the meaning of normality, and Ryan's future would play out in the courtroom in Indiana that fall. The October ruling that followed the September 19 case conference marked the completion of the initial administrative steps in Ryan's case. Soon thereafter, Vaughan filed a formal appeal with the Indiana Department of Education (IDOE).[59] The first IDOE hearing, held on November 1, revealed the tensions at the heart of the Ryan White saga. During the hearing, Vaughan sparred with special education expert Justin O'Brien, who had been called as a witness by WSC attorneys. When Vaughan questioned O'Brien's credentials, O'Brien exploded. "We're endangering the lives of children based on incomplete information, and you damn well know it," he exclaimed as he slapped the court bench for maximum effect. In a similarly heated exchange, WSC lawyers tried unsuccessfully to force one of Vaughan's witnesses, the head of the ISBH's communicable disease division, to admit that "health officials do not know with certainty how AIDS is spread."[60] Though the WSC's legal team fell short in this respect, it also submitted over thirty "medical articles which attempted to highlight . . . the unknown matters concerning the disease." Sensing that Vaughan and the Whites had won the epidemiological argument during the November 1 IDOE hearing, however, the WSC's attorneys decided to emphasize "Ryan's best interests" in their post-hearing brief.[61] According to the WSC legal team, given Ryan's interlocking disabilities, an "'appropriate' education" delivered through "homebound instruction"—supplemented with "visits by friends and classmates"—would best "serve . . . Ryan's academic needs." Ryan's hemophilia and AIDS precluded "education in the regular classroom," the WSC attorneys insisted, whereas "homebound instruction" would offer "consistency and continuity in academic instruction," since Ryan could "participate by telephone four times more often than he is able to go to school." These legal arguments affirmed Ryan's status as a sickly, disabled child while ostensibly prioritizing "continuity in his education" and socialization—in other words, normality.[62]

The IDOE hearing officer, Kathleen Madinger Angelone, was not convinced. She ruled in Ryan's favor in late November, dismissing the WSC's epidemiological claims while asserting that "continuity of the Child's education must be assured" and that "the Child is able to perform adequately in the regular classroom setting."[63] By paving the way for Ryan's return to school, Angelone gave Ryan what he called "a great birthday present" ahead of his fourteenth birthday on December 6.[64] "Yea! Great! I'm going back to school," Ryan cheered when he learned the news. "The biggest thing in his life is school," lawyer Charles Vaughan noted, again underlining Ryan's desire for normality.[65] "But," Tom Brokaw told *Nightly News* viewers in the wake of the IDOE decision, "the controversy is still far from over."[66] School officials and many parents obviously disagreed with the IDOE ruling, but it was unclear whether the WSC would appeal, given its mounting legal fees.[67] The decision to appeal or not to appeal required the approval of the entire school board, so several weeks passed before the decision came down.[68] Eventually, in a December 17 meeting that the *Kokomo Tribune* dubbed a "media

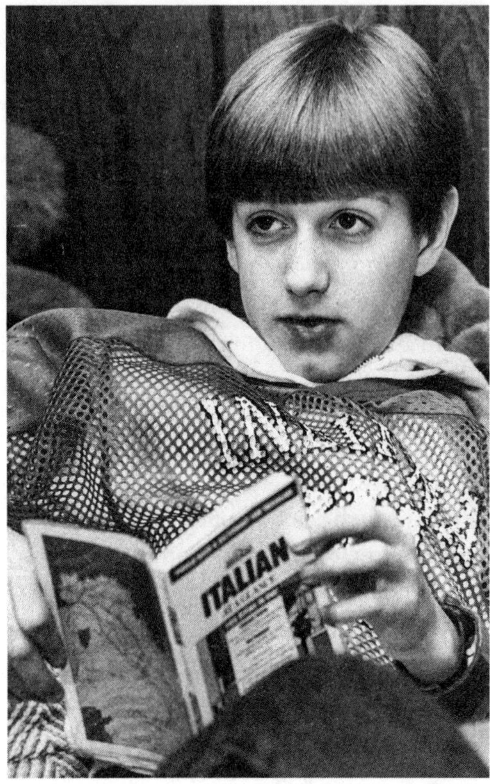

Clad in an Indiana University jersey, Ryan White brushes up on his Italian before heading to Rome in early 1986. Howard County Historical Society, Kokomo, IN.

event," the Western School Board agreed to appeal Angelone's ruling. Just as others had justified their opposition to Ryan's campaign, the school board supported its decision by pointing to lingering questions about AIDS and the transmission of HIV. "The puzzle of AIDS is incomplete," school board president Dan Carter proclaimed, thus coining a slogan of sorts for those campaigning to keep Ryan out of WMS.[69]

RYAN IN ROME

The appeals board hearing would take place on February 6, 1986. In the meantime, as the Whites celebrated the Christmas holiday and marked the end of a "hectic" year, Ryan's status as an international celebrity was solidified.[70] In what the *Kokomo Tribune* described as an early Christmas gift, the Italian state television station RAI (Radiotelevisione Italiana) announced that it would fly Ryan, Jeanne, and Andrea White to Rome, where the family would appear on the program *Italia Sera*.[71] A US-based RAI representative told the *Los Angeles Times* that Italians were "interested in the problem of AIDS and the panic around it. They want to talk to Ryan about being in the middle of this for a year now—the social aspects of it."[72] According to Jeanne White, Ryan also received Christmas greetings, gifts, and cards "from Japan, Ecuador and places I've never heard of." "AIDS Victim Now a Celebrity," a January 1986 *Chicago Tribune* headline read.[73]

Once in Rome and on the set of *Italia Sera*, the slight young globetrotter from Kokomo "won the hearts of viewers," as UPI put it, and even spurred one family from the town of Gorgonzola "to invite that fabulous boy to come and visit us."[74] Through their appearance on Italian TV, Jeanne White hoped "to show the world another side of AIDS," while Ryan sought to "inform people about AIDS and tell them really not to be afraid of AIDS."[75] Ryan also expressed his desire to return to school. "I hope they let me back," said Ryan, who wore a plaid button-down shirt and a dark tie on the broadcast. "I want to be treated like a normal person."[76]

The Whites' trip to Rome not only revealed how normality and a particular understanding of education shaped the Ryan White saga but also spoke to Ryan's exceptional status in the world of AIDS. Ryan's youthful charm, nonthreatening sexuality, and "innocence" distinguished him from other people with AIDS and transformed him into an international ambassador and educator on HIV/AIDS issues. As news media, public, and political interest in the Ryan White case grew in 1986 and beyond, so too did Ryan's celebrity and legend.

CHAPTER THREE

AIDS VICTIM NOW A CELEBRITY

Boy, celebrity life must be tough, huh?

Debbie, letter to Ryan White, January 31, 1989

The White family had never seen anything like it. An "overflowing media pool" greeted them upon their arrival from Rome on February 5, 1986, the evening before an Indiana Department of Education appeals board would determine whether Ryan could return to Western Middle School. "The media literally took up a whole wing of the airport," Jeanne White told the *Kokomo Tribune*. This horde of reporters and camerapersons had converged on the Indianapolis International Airport to obtain footage of, and perhaps a statement from, Ryan White—the sickly Kokomo teenager plucked from obscurity and catapulted into a curious kind of superstardom. After a long trip back from Italy, though, Ryan was exhausted, airsick, and in considerable pain due to some bleeding in his elbow, so he scurried through the airport—past shouting reporters and flashing cameras—without providing a comment. After navigating their way out of the airport, the Whites returned to their home in south Kokomo to find a telegram from President Ronald Reagan and his wife, Nancy, wishing Ryan a belated happy birthday.[1]

Ryan was a celebrity, in large part because of the courtroom drama that had defined his life for the past half year. But while Ryan's legal saga would soon come to a close, his fame would enter a new, more intense phase beginning in 1986. By that point, nearly five years after the initial Centers for Disease Control and Prevention reports concerning Pneumocystis carinii pneumonia among gay men, the AIDS epidemic had no clear spokesperson or "poster child," despite the best efforts of activists such as Bobbi Campbell and the People with AIDS collective.[2] That would all change when Ryan emerged victorious in his legal and public relations battle against the Western School Corporation in the first half of 1986. This triumph further cemented Ryan White's status as a celebrity spokesperson, a "poster boy" who could demystify and educate the public about AIDS.

But because Ryan was not necessarily a typical person with AIDS—given his age, sexuality, and "squeaky-clean" image—his visibility in the world of AIDS crowded out other populations more closely associated with the illness (especially men who had sex with men and intravenous drug users). He was not even a particularly representative *child* with HIV/AIDS, given the epidemic's disproportionate impact on Black and Brown youth.[3] Further, his story's focus on awareness and acceptance also helped entrench what Cindy Patton calls the "national pedagogy" on AIDS, which revolved around narrow questions concerning the transmission of HIV and the need for greater tolerance of PWAS. By reducing a complex public health emergency to an issue of personal responsibility, morality, and kindness, these questions reinforced the epidemic's "hierarchies of victimhood," which placed "blameless" PWAS over those who had contracted HIV through sex or intravenous drug use, white PWAS over Black and Brown PWAS, and enlightened, open-minded members of the "general public" over those who discriminated against PWAS.[4]

POSTER BOY(S)

On account of his youth, race, heterosexuality, and perceived innocence, Ryan White became the most famous person with AIDS in the country (if not the world) in the mid-1980s. Ryan captured national and international headlines after he was barred from attending his middle school in July 1985. Unlike other PWAS, Ryan was immediately embraced by the media and the public. Ordinary people sent messages of love and support from across the country and around the globe. Around the same time, the public had learned of actor Rock Hudson's AIDS diagnosis. Together, the Hudson and White cases intensified concerns that AIDS might be "spreading" beyond the marginalized communities in which it was once believed to be localized—namely injecting drug users and MSM.[5] What was previously a public health crisis among certain stigmatized populations alone now seemed to threaten the "general public."[6] In this moment, Ryan came to symbolize the plight of normal, presumably innocent people with AIDS, and his struggle to return to school came to represent a broader struggle against ignorance, fear, and closed-mindedness. Just as Ryan White had served as a "poster boy" for the Howard County Hemophilia Society back in 1973, he emerged as *the* face of AIDS—and a particular type of AIDS education—in the mid- to late 1980s.[7]

There could have been other poster boys, though. Instead of dismissing or ignoring the suspicious deaths of disproportionately Black and Brown sex workers and drug users in the 1960s and 1970s, medical officials might have alerted the press about a mysterious new illness affecting vulnerable populations.[8] Instead of waiting for a "sympathetic" PWA like Ryan to help raise awareness about AIDS, and instead of maligning the groups most devastated by the epidemic, elected officials and mainstream media outlets could have elevated the Black, Brown, and queer activists working to address the crisis in the early 1980s. The often-overlooked stories of Robert Rayford, Bobbi Campbell, and countless injecting drug users who contracted HIV help illuminate what was hidden and what was lost.

The virus now known as HIV has lived in human bodies since at least the early twentieth century.[9] Researchers have determined that 1920s Kinshasa (in what is now the Democratic Republic of the Congo) served as a key site in the early transmission of HIV.[10] In subsequent decades, HIV and AIDS made several suspected appearances in North America and Western Europe. As Mirko Grmek documented in 1990, over a dozen cases detailed "in American medical journals between early 1940 and June 5, 1981 (when the CDC announced their observations of Pneumocystis pneumonia in homosexuals) . . . fit the present clinical definition of AIDS."[11]

Scientists generally identify Robert Rayford (1953–69) as the first person to die of AIDS-related causes in the United States. A Black teenager who never left his hometown of St. Louis, Rayford may have contracted HIV while performing sex work, or he may have been sexually assaulted by someone carrying the virus. After he fell ill at the age of thirteen or fourteen, Rayford experienced unusual swelling in his legs, torso, and genitalia.[12] As the *Chicago Tribune*'s John Crewdson wrote in 1987, Rayford had "grown thin and pale, fatigued and short of breath."[13] Eventually, young Robert checked himself into St. Louis's City Hospital, but it didn't do much good. "Baffled" by Rayford's symptoms, the doctors there treated their patient as an oddity and a commodity. They "poked and prodded and photographed him for their archives," extracting and exploiting while offering little in the way of care apart from antibiotics. Although doctors knew that Robert's immune system had stopped functioning properly, they couldn't explain why, nor could they help him fend off the opportunistic infections that threatened him. After Robert Rayford died on May 16, 1969, the pathologist who performed his autopsy discovered a set of purplish lesions denoting Kaposi's sarcoma, a rare form of cancer that would become intimately associated with AIDS in the 1980s.[14]

Despite the aggressive and mysterious nature of Robert's illness, it triggered no significant news media coverage, meaning that the medical professionals who studied his condition failed, or refused, to notify the public or the press. The available evidence also indicates that these doctors neglected to reach out to those in St. Louis's depressed Old North neighborhood, where Robert Rayford lived. Doing so might have helped determine how Rayford had gotten sick and whether any of his neighbors were exhibiting similar symptoms. But the same historical processes that had condemned Rayford to live in abject poverty—white supremacy, racial segregation, capital flight—all but ensured that he would die in anonymity and that the disease that killed him would live on, infecting and draining the life from other bodies on the margins.[15] As Jih-Fei Cheng writes, Robert's illness and death "did not prompt the same public alarm as arrived just over a decade later, when doctors began to notice signs of Kaposi's sarcoma among primarily white, middle-class gay men" in New York City, San Francisco, and Los Angeles.[16] Not until 1987, when Western blot testing on tissue samples extracted from Rayford's body confirmed his HIV infection, would the public learn of Rayford.[17] Even then—around the same time that historian of science Evelynn Hammonds expressed her shock concerning "the extent and rate" at which AIDS was spreading among Black Americans—news of Rayford's illness did not unsettle dominant conceptions of AIDS as a "white man's disease."[18] Rayford's story thus joined those of countless other Black and Brown PWAs—and their kinship networks—which have been forgotten, discarded, lost.[19] Robert Rayford did not become a poster child.[20]

Neither did the injecting drug users who began contracting HIV during the mid- to late seventies.[21] In New York City—where a fiscal crisis had fueled neoliberal economic restructuring, and anxieties about crime, drugs, and disorder had compelled elected officials to "get tough"—the pervasive intravenous use of heroin and cocaine led to the rapid spread of HIV in the late 1970s and early 1980s.[22] Restrictions on access to sterile needles and other injection equipment exacerbated the crisis, which remains the largest known HIV outbreak in injecting drug users in human history.[23] In response to this epidemic, intravenous drug users in New York City adopted safer injection practices, reducing syringe sharing and increasing the availability and use of sterile injection equipment. With the legalization of needle-exchange programs in the early 1990s, the New York State Department of Health—in coordination with New York City–based activists and the city government—began funding and issuing licenses for such programs. These measures helped to dramatically curb the spread of HIV among people who injected drugs.[24] Nevertheless, intravenous drug users garnered little sympathy from the public in the 1970s—when their deaths were often derisively blamed on the "junkie flu" or the "dwindles"—or at the height of the HIV/AIDS crisis in the 1980s and 1990s.[25]

Bobbi Campbell had struggled mightily to become a household name. As the self-proclaimed "AIDS poster boy," Campbell sought to raise awareness about the illness following his diagnosis in October 1981.[26] A white, openly gay registered nurse living in San Francisco, Campbell achieved some success in his campaign, no doubt because of his effervescent personality, good looks, whiteness, and connection to the medical establishment. Unlike Robert Rayford and countless other people on the margins who contracted HIV in the final decades of the twentieth century, Bobbi Campbell attained a certain level of visibility, which allowed him to raise awareness about the AIDS epidemic. Campbell appeared on national television and graced the cover of *Newsweek* magazine, reaching "the pinnacle of AIDS consciousness," as one admirer put it in 1984.[27] "The biggest news of the year," Bobbi Campbell wrote in his diary in 1983, "is that BOBBY [Hilliard, his partner] & I ARE ON THE COVER OF NEWSWEEK. Too much. He looks handsome and worried and I look handsome and defiant, clutching him."[28] "Gay America," the cover read, "Sex, Politics and the Impact of AIDS."[29] Under the aegis of the People with AIDS collective, Campbell also cowrote (with fellow AIDS activist Michael Callen, among others) the influential Denver Principles, which advised against the use of the word "victim" to describe PWAs.[30]

In one way, Campbell's successes were short-lived. He has largely been forgotten since his death in August 1984, just four months before Ryan White's AIDS diagnosis and approximately a year before White became a household name. In another way, though, his activism helped advance cultural perceptions of AIDS as both a "white man's disease" and a "gay plague." These two ideas had begun to take hold with the CDC's initial reports on Kaposi's sarcoma in white middle-class gay men during the early 1980s, and they proliferated throughout the decade. Ryan White's story, with which so many Americans and others around the world became familiar starting in 1985, challenged the widely held notion that HIV and AIDS exclusively (or almost exclusively) afflicted gay men. But it also fortified the "hierarchy of victimhood" that placed young PWAs with hemophilia over those who had contracted HIV through sex or injection drug use.[31] Further, his story did little to dislodge the idea that AIDS was a "white" epidemic. Ryan's growing visibility in the second half of the 1980s ensured that AIDS would remain a white story, even as the epidemic increasingly ravaged communities of color.

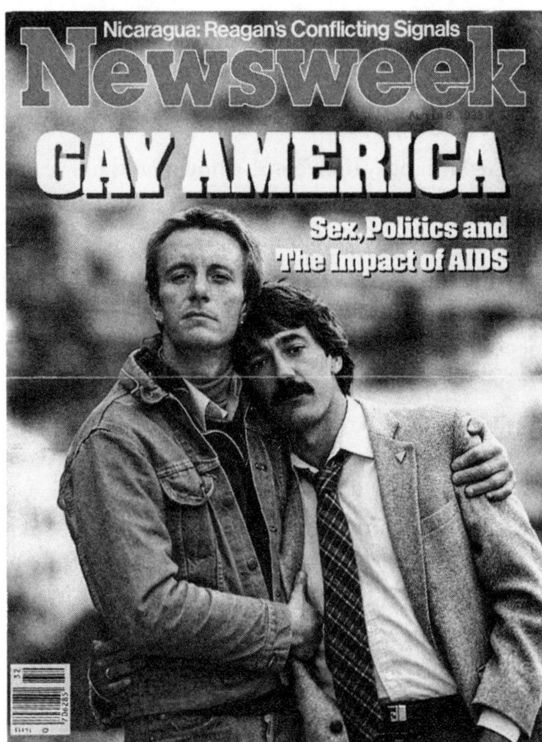
Nicaragua: Reagan's Conflicting Signals

Newsweek

GAY AMERICA

Sex, Politics and The Impact of AIDS

Bobbi Campbell (*left*) and Bobby Hilliard on the cover of *Newsweek* magazine, August 8, 1983. Digital resource published by the Regents of the University of California. Special Collections, University of California, San Francisco Libraries, Online Archive of California.

FULL COURT PRESS

While national news outlets had diligently covered the Ryan White saga since J. O. Smith decided to bar Ryan from Western Middle School in the summer of 1985, their coverage grew more frequent and intense as Ryan's courtroom drama reached a crescendo in early 1986. Each of the "Big Three" nightly news broadcasts ran multiple stories about Ryan White in February 1986, when the State Board of Special Education Appeals ruled that the teenager could return to school if he received medical clearance from Howard County's public health officer, Dr. Alan Adler. Although Adler later recalled that those in the county's public health department "felt that it was probably safe" for Ryan to return to WMS—based on the independent research they had conducted on HIV/AIDS—he also consulted with several other medical professionals, including the head of Indiana University's Medical Center and Ryan's chief physician, Dr. Martin Kleiman. These experts all assured Adler that Ryan could attend WMS without endangering the health and safety of his schoolmates, teachers, or himself.[32]

Given the widespread public interest in Ryan's case, Adler announced his decision during a televised news conference, held shortly after he performed a brief medical examination on Ryan.[33] Before a row of television cameras in an unremarkable county government building, Adler explained that Ryan White's "present medical condition is such that he should not pose any threat to his fellow students, teachers and others." Ryan was heading back to school, and the whole world knew it. But even though Ryan "ha[d] the full right" to attend classes in person the next day, Adler requested a one-week delay, in part because of a surge in flu cases at WMS and in part because school officials could use some additional time to prepare for Ryan's return.[34]

During that week, the White family traveled to New York City for an appearance on NBC's *Today Show* and the *CBS Morning News*.[35] After the Whites returned to Indiana, they collaborated with the Howard County Health Department and the Western School Corporation on a set of precautionary guidelines designed "to facilitate the re-enrollment of the AIDS/ARC child to the school setting."[36] These guidelines were excessive, to say the least, and completely out of step with the scientific consensus on HIV/AIDS. Their main purpose, however, was "to dispel a lot of [the] fears" swirling around Kokomo and Russiaville at the time related to the communicability of the virus.[37] Ryan would use separate bathroom facilities ("which should be cleaned daily by the prescribed method"), eat with "single service disposable . . . utensils," and toss his trash in a separate bin, the contents of which would be double-bagged and incinerated.[38]

With these precautionary (yet unnecessary) measures in place, Ryan White returned to school on the morning of Friday, February 21, 1986. Reporters and television cameras were prohibited from entering Western Middle School that day, but that didn't deter members of the press corps from camping out in the snow.[39] According to the *Indianapolis Star*, "at least" fifty journalists, photographers, and camerapersons waited outside. The media presence was so overwhelming that school officials opened up a "special waiting area" for news media personnel at the adjacent Western Elementary School.[40] By most accounts, Ryan's experience during his first day back was pleasant and relatively uneventful. "It was a lot of fun," he noted in a media scrum immediately after the final school bell had rung. "I'm glad to be back." When asked how his fellow students had treated him, Ryan responded, "Just like anybody else."[41] And when asked what he was "looking forward to now," he replied, "Well, getting back to normal life."[42] For at least a moment, then, Ryan's life seemed relatively normal, and he wanted things to stay that way.

But news media dispatches also spotlighted the community's formidable opposition to Ryan's return. Braving the wintry conditions, a small group of students from Western High School picketed outside of WMS. One of the high schoolers, Don Hochstedler—wearing aviator-style sunglasses and sporting a hair-metal hairdo—carried a sign that read, "STUDENTS AGAINST AIDS." In a clip that aired on the *CBS Evening News*, Hochstedler declared, "I ain't got nothing against Ryan or anything. I just don't want AIDS in our school."[43] Yet as ABC's Jerry King noted on *World News Tonight*, this "small, brief demonstration against Ryan's return to classes" paled in comparison to "the main protest," which "took the form of absenteeism."[44] WMS principal Ron Colby had expected the "absentee rate" to be "a little higher than normal" on the day that Ryan returned to school.[45] It was not. A staggering 42 percent of the student body stayed home that day "to avoid being exposed to the fourteen-year-old victim of AIDS," as reporter Jim Cummins put it on *NBC Nightly News*.[46] Cummins's story then featured Allen and Kathy Shepherd, whose four children had "stayed at home and watched television" at their parents' behest. "It's a deadly disease, and I don't want to take that chance with my children," Allen Shepherd explained to a gaggle of reporters. "If he sneezes or anything, kids can get it," the eldest Shepherd daughter asserted matter-of-factly but incorrectly.[47] The community's opposition to Ryan's February 21 return to WMS—depicted in stark detail in newspapers and on the nightly news—cast negative light on the residents of Kokomo and Russiaville.

So too did parents' successful appeal for a temporary injunction barring White from school on the same day he had returned to WMS. Several members of the Concerned Citizens and Parents of Children Attending Western School Corporation organization filed a petition for a temporary restraining order in Howard County Circuit Court.[48] Judge R. Alan Brubaker ruled in favor of the petitioners on the afternoon of February 21, transforming what was a joyous and fairly smooth return to classes into an unmitigated disaster for Ryan and his family.[49] "They welcomed him back, and they gave him a good time today, and I think it's very wrong to take that away from him right now," Jeanne White told viewers of ABC's *World News Tonight*.[50]

While those who sought the injunction against Ryan—"angry parents," as *NBC Nightly News* characterized them—celebrated Brubaker's decision, they simultaneously undermined their cause by fiendishly cheering after the

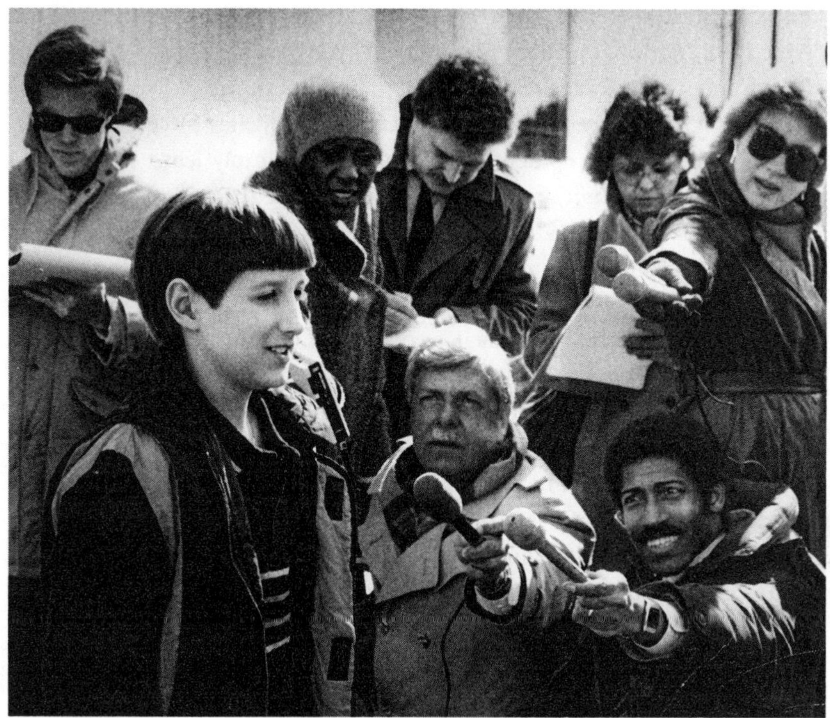

Ryan White addresses reporters following his return to Western Middle School, February 21, 1986. Howard County Historical Society, Kokomo, IN.

judge issued his ruling.[51] As the *Kokomo Tribune* described it, "The city had been moderately successful in weathering a generally negative opinion the rest of the country apparently had of Kokomo—until Feb. 21. That day . . . a local judge slapped a restraining order on [Ryan's] return to school. But what appeared to enrage a national television news audience more than the decision was that school patrons who sought the injunction left the courtroom cheering and flashing thumbs-up [signs]." A swift backlash ensued. "Ryan White has put Kokomo [pop. 45,500] on the national media map," Rogers Worthington wrote in an early draft of one of his *Chicago Tribune* articles. "And Kokomo . . . is none too happy with the limelight and a national image it sees as one of unsophisticated bully." As the *Kokomo Tribune* put it, "Almost immediately" after the February 21 hearing, "generally hostile letters from around the nation flooded the city."[52]

These letters and other responses spoke not only to the high-profile nature of Ryan White's legal saga but also to the solidification of a broad cultural narrative concerning HIV/AIDS awareness, which Cindy Patton has termed the "national pedagogy" on AIDS.[53] As Ryan's celebrity grew alongside coverage of the resistance he faced in his community, Kokomo became increasingly synonymous with ignorance, one of the key forces supposedly driving the HIV/AIDS epidemic. If locals could simply learn more about AIDS and treat Ryan with respect and kindness, the thinking went, then all would be well. As Ryan White became the most famous PWA in the United States (and perhaps the world) in the latter half of the 1980s, he also became the face of this national pedagogy, which prioritized individual over collective action and fortified the racial, sexual, class, and other hierarchies that defined the AIDS epidemic in the United States.

This pedagogical narrative proliferated in the days after Brubaker's decision. For instance, it informed the letter that Mike Hippler sent to Western Middle School's student body president on February 24. "If you would only read a little bit [and] educate yourselves, you would learn that Ryan poses no threat to you," wrote Hippler, who worked for the San Francisco–based gay and lesbian publication the *Bay Area Reporter*.[54] (Hippler would die of AIDS-related causes in 1991.) Similarly, in a letter published in the *Kokomo Tribune* just days after Brubaker's ruling, another San Franciscan named Jeff Hayward described the "hysteria" whipped up "by those who refuse to accept information other than what they choose to believe." Hayward further reprimanded locals in Kokomo and Russiaville "for needlessly hounding an innocent young person at a time when he most needs support."[55] The *New York Times* editorial board advanced this narrative as well, casting Ryan as a "normal" PWA who was paying the price for Kokomo's ignorance. "Ryan White, a normal Indiana kid except that he has AIDS, is being kept out of school because some adults aren't learning about the disease fast enough," the board members wrote on February 27.[56]

These examples reflected Ryan White's unique position in the world of AIDS as an exceptional, "normal," "innocent," and increasingly famous PWA. They also suggested that Ryan would play a key role in developing the national pedagogy on AIDS. As more and more Americans learned of Ryan's plight, they absorbed the primary lesson of his story as it was presented in dominant news media and popular narratives: the HIV/AIDS crisis could be mitigated through greater compassion and awareness among those who were not at high risk of infection. As innocuous as this lesson seemed, it nevertheless reinforced the epidemic's "hierarchies of victimhood" and widened the perceived gap between those who were living with HIV/AIDS and those who were not.

"I KNOW YOU"

Ryan's increasing visibility was bad news for Kokomo and Russiaville. The temporary injunction granted by Judge Brubaker in February 1986 had engendered even more public sympathy for Ryan White while stoking outrage against the Concerned Citizens and Parents group and others throughout the Kokomo area. The following month, March 1986, Kokomo's mayor, Stephen Daily, detailed the "growing frustration in the people in Kokomo as they watch the national media cover the events here."[57] At the time, local Baptist minister Ruth Lawson later recalled, Daily "was just so disturbed about the negative image of Kokomo" developing in the popular press.[58] Seeking to offset the bad publicity generated by the White controversy, Kokomo's leaders even set out to launch "a citywide fund drive to benefit AIDS research."[59] According to *Kokomo Tribune* staff writer Christopher M. MacNeil, "The proposed benefit is Mayor Stephen J. Daily's strategy to blunt the public image beating the city has taken because of local reaction to Ryan White's fight for a classroom education."[60]

When that fight came to an abrupt conclusion in the spring of 1986, it made the resistance to Ryan's return seem all the more futile and foolish. In April, a circuit judge in Clinton County, Indiana, overturned the temporary injunction requested by parents in neighboring Howard County. Ryan was once again allowed to attend classes in person at Western Middle School. Though some parents in and around Kokomo pursued an appeal, their case had little chance of succeeding, and it was ultimately dismissed in July of that year.[61] But immediately after Ryan returned to WMS in April, his most ardent opponents—a cohort of twenty-one sixth- and seventh-graders and their parents—launched an entirely new school to avoid interacting with the young boy with AIDS. Their "makeshift schoolhouse," reporter Anthony Mason explained on the April 22 edition of the *CBS Evening News*, "was hurriedly set up in an old American Legion Hall" to serve "as a refuge for students from the Western Middle School just a few miles away."[62] Mason's report revealed the lengths to which some parents would go to protect their children. Given the fact that Ryan posed no threat to his classmates, however, and given the poor optics of segregated education (just a decade or two after some of the most visible and contentious battles over school integration and busing), such coverage could only have shed further negative light on Kokomo.

As Kokomo's stock fell, Ryan's rose. In the weeks following the Clinton County Circuit Court decision on April 9, Ryan and his family embarked on something of a publicity tour, which confirmed Ryan's status as not only a celebrity but also *the* face of HIV/AIDS awareness. Immediately after the court ruling, Ryan decided to return to school, passing up a trip to Los Angeles and an appearance on *The Tonight Show Starring Johnny Carson*.[63] But later that month, at the invitation of Olympic diver Greg Louganis, Ryan and his mother made a quick trip down to Indianapolis, site of the national platform diving championships. There, Louganis—the reigning national champion—successfully defended his title before giving his gold medal to Ryan. The encounter made national headlines and kindled a friendship that would last until Ryan's death in 1990. "I couldn't believe how difficult the people in Kokomo were making it for Ryan," Louganis told the *Indianapolis Star* in 1987. "I have a lot to learn from him. I think a lot of people do."[64]

Days after the diving competition, Ryan flew out to New York City to be interviewed on ABC's *Good Morning America* and to attend a benefit for the American Foundation for AIDS Research (better known as amfAR). On *Good Morning America*, Ryan and Jeanne stressed the importance of raising awareness about HIV's modes of transmission. Asked about "the gang that didn't go back" to Western Middle School because Ryan was now attending classes there, Ryan remarked, "I can see [that] they're scared, but with all the facts, I don't really see why."[65] Backstage in the *Good Morning America* green room, actor Tom Cruise spotted Ryan and stated, "I know you. You're Ryan White." Ryan would serve as a guest of honor at the lavish amfAR benefit, held several days later at the Jacob Javits Center and cohosted by actress Elizabeth Taylor and fashion designer Calvin Klein. At the gala, Jeanne and Ryan (clad in a tuxedo) rubbed shoulders with Yoko Ono and New York mayor Ed Koch, while Andy Warhol snapped photographs of the mother-son duo. Perry Ellis, Brooke Shields, Donna Karan, Oscar de la Renta, Paul Simon, and many other VIPs were also in attendance.[66]

By February of the next year (a month before the formation of ACT UP), Indiana's health commissioner, Woodrow Myers Jr., could confidently assert that "Ryan White is the best known AIDS victim in the United States if not the world"—and one who posed "the lowest possible political risk" for elected officials seeking to address the epidemic. Myers made these comments in a letter to Mark Lubbers, an executive assistant to Indiana's Republican governor, Robert D. Orr. Lubbers was scheduled to meet later that week with Mitch Daniels, then serving as the White House director of political and intergovernmental affairs and a political advisor to President Reagan. In his letter, Myers offered Lubbers some talking points concerning the

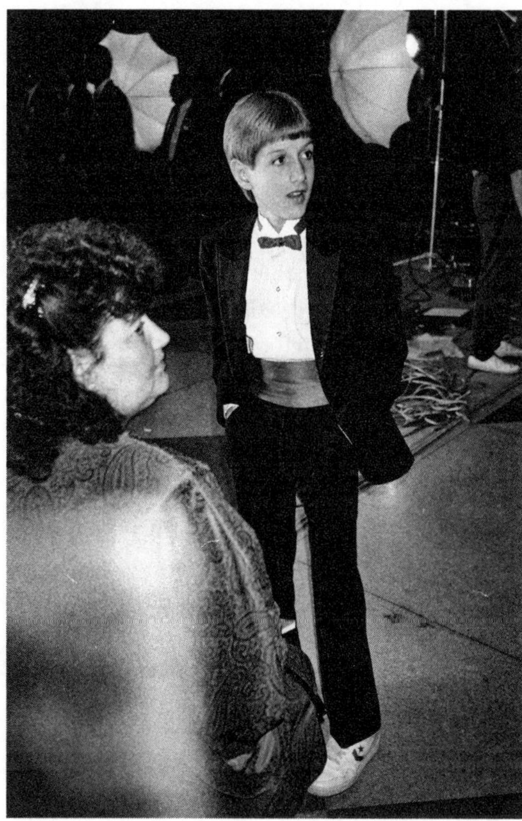

Photographic reproduction from Andy Warhol's 35mm negative. Ryan White and his mother Jeanne White at To Care Is to Cure at Javits Center, 1986. Image and Artwork © 2023 The Andy Warhol Foundation for the Visual Arts, Inc. / Licensed by ARS.

Reagan administration's failure to adequately confront the HIV/AIDS crisis. "The Reagans have not had a strong public presence on the AIDS issue," Myers wrote, in stark contrast to "their very strong presence on the drug abuse issue." Myers was no doubt referring to the president's intensification of the war on drugs and Nancy Reagan's infamous "Just Say No" campaign. By singing Ryan and Jeanne's praises in his letter to Lubbers, Myers hoped to offer the Reagans an opportunity to become more involved on AIDS. "Ryan and his mother are friendly, pleasingly shy and very 'Hoosier,'" he explained, pointing to the Whites as the epitome of "midwestern nice." "They have been involved in AIDS educational activities throughout the state, in other states and overseas," Myers continued. He then proposed a "public event with the Whites and the Reagans," which "would serve to recognize [Ryan's] bravery, applaud the White's [*sic*] willingness to help other Hoosiers understand this disease and to encourage Americans to come forward both to educate others and to learn."[67] Myers's letter testified to Ryan's growing visibility and his key role in promulgating the national pedagogy on AIDS.

Lubbers seemed intrigued by Myers's suggestion. He likely discussed the proposal with Daniels at dinner and then followed up with him in a letter later that month. "If the President is interested in this issue at all, this would be a terrific way to punctuate the federal government's initiatives—whatever they are," Lubbers wrote, seemingly unable to define the nature of the federal response to HIV/AIDS. "A Ryan White visit coterminously would be the best insulation you could have against civil rights zealots on the left and moral zealots on the right," Lubbers's letter continued. "This is just a poor kid from Kokomo with hemophilia who got bad blood in a transfusion." Lubbers thus recognized Ryan's potential political utility as a well-known, innocent, and nearly unassailable "poor kid" with AIDS. But although the Reagans had connected with Ryan before—via that telegram sent in early 1986—the "First Family event" suggested by Myers and apparently endorsed by Lubbers never materialized.[68] Still, these high-level political discussions demonstrated just how brilliantly Ryan's star shone at this moment—and how his stardom would be marshaled in the service of a particular type of AIDS pedagogy and politics.

MOVING ON

Despite Ryan's legal victory, his return to "normal school," and his budding friendships with Louganis and pop superstars Michael Jackson and Elton John, he still faced difficulties at school and with his health.[69] His eighth-grade year at Western High School began normally enough—the national news coverage notwithstanding—but it was soon marred by trips to the hospital and harassment at school and in town.[70] In the spring of 1987, frustrated by the situation in Kokomo and Russiaville, the White family decamped for Cicero, a small Hamilton County town approximately thirty miles south of Kokomo. (Elton John loaned the family the money to purchase their home there.) Considering Ryan's celebrity status, the family's escape from Kokomo—and subsequent embrace by the people of the Cicero area—would be covered extensively in the press and in the made-for-TV film *The Ryan White Story*. Shortly after Ryan had arrived in Cicero—and before he had formally enrolled at Hamilton Heights High School in nearby Arcadia—he appeared on the cover of *People* magazine. The cover story, and White's remarks therein, portrayed Kokomo in a particularly harsh light.

"Ryan White is 15, and he is dying," the piece began. "His school kicked him out. Townspeople slashed the tires on the family car and pelted it with eggs; schoolmates taunted him; someone fired a bullet [actually a BB pellet] through the living-room window." On account of these conditions, Ryan told *People*, "I didn't want to die there [in Kokomo]. I really didn't want to be buried there."[71]

The entire country and, indeed, the world watched in August 1987 as Ryan White enrolled at Hamilton Heights. There, he received a warm welcome "in sharp contrast to what happened to him last year when he tried to go to school in nearby Kokomo," NBC's Jim Cummins reported on the *Nightly News*.[72] National news outlets from NBC to the Associated Press emphasized Ryan's new lease on life following his move to Cicero and underscored the importance of education and "heightened awareness" in facilitating Ryan's "smooth transition" to Hamilton Heights.[73] "We've looked at it objectively and looked at the facts," the school's principal, Tony Cook, stated on the *Nightly News*. "Most of us have made up our minds philosophically that Ryan's no threat to us physically."[74] Cook also told the Associated Press that "the knowledge of the disease here is very high, so the majority are objective and open-minded."[75]

Just a few months later, with the fall semester wrapping up, Governor Robert Orr bestowed Indiana's highest civic honor, the Sagamore of the Wabash, upon Ryan and Jeanne White for their efforts to raise awareness about HIV/AIDS. Hamilton Heights students too received recognition from the governor for their compassion and tolerance.[76] Reporting on the ceremony at which Orr presented these awards, ABC's Peter Jennings explained, "Thanks to Ryan's doggedness in talking about AIDS, the country as a whole has a little clearer picture about AIDS and society." Jennings also took the opportunity to praise the news media for its coverage of the White saga, which had boosted Ryan's profile and bolstered his cause. "We are sometimes not very proud of the media circus which we impose on people's private lives," Jennings admitted. "And yet if there hadn't been all the national fuss when Ryan was first kept out of school, perhaps people in other places would not have been so motivated to learn the facts about AIDS and to act as they did."[77] Ryan's highly publicized move from Kokomo to Cicero thus reflected a supposed national reckoning on AIDS, a pivot from ignorance and fear to education and acceptance.

Accordingly, the distinction between Kokomo and Cicero served a key function in the dominant Ryan White story and the national pedagogy it supported. This distinction between the towns shaped Ryan's March 1988 testimony before the President's Commission on the HIV Epidemic in Washington, DC. "My battle has been against AIDS and the discrimination surrounding it," the youngster noted. "Eventually, I won the right to attend school, but the prejudice was still there" in the Western School Corporation and the wider community. Now "we feel we have a home, a supportive school, and lots of friends," Ryan proclaimed. "I'm just one of the kids, and all because the students at Hamilton Heights High School listened to the facts, educated their parents and themselves, and believed in me." His testimony concluded with a ringing endorsement of HIV/AIDS education. "Hamilton Heights High School is proof that AIDS education in schools works," Ryan declared.[78] White sounded similar notes in his July 1988 address at the annual convention of the National Education Association. "Teachers can play an important role in helping an AIDS student be accepted and treated as normal as possible by teaching the facts, not the myths," Ryan told the 8,000 delegates gathered in New Orleans. "By proper education, AIDS can be a disease, not a dirty word."[79]

An October 1988 documentary program geared toward educating children about AIDS revealed how Ryan's Hamilton Heights classmates, through their kindness and a concerted awareness campaign, had enabled the youngster's pursuit of "normality." Titled *I Have AIDS: A Teenager's Story*, the program was distributed via the Children's Television Workshop and Public Broadcasting Service. It opens on Ryan, clad in a bright yellow T-shirt, his hair poofy, his face swollen. "I'm Ryan White, I'm sixteen years old, and I have AIDS," he states, looking directly into the camera. In keeping with the dominant narrative of the Ryan White saga, the documentary draws a contrast between Ryan's treatment at the Western schools and Hamilton Heights High School and proposes "education" and "awareness" as antidotes to the AIDS crisis. At Hamilton Heights, the narrator indicates, "Ryan was accepted as part of the gang, mostly because before he even got there, the school set up a special AIDS education program so everyone in the school—kids and teachers—learned as much as they could about Ryan's disease." The documentary also underlines how seamlessly Ryan fit in at Hamilton Heights High School. One of the students featured in the documentary tells a reporter, "He has AIDS, sure, but we've accepted that. He's just another one of the guys!" A young woman similarly notes, "I think he's just like everyone else." Such framing allowed Ryan to seem "normal," despite his AIDS and "celebrity" status, both of which are referenced in the program.[80]

These sorts of cultural artifacts not only testified to Ryan's fame and visibility but also reflected and shaped prevailing conceptions of the HIV/

AIDS epidemic. By positioning Ryan as an exceptional yet normal PWA—the courageous, "innocent" boy next door who hung out with the likes of NFL star Howie Long and actor Charlie Sheen—news media and other popular accounts diverted attention away from other PWAs, especially queer people and people of color. In so doing, these accounts shored up the interlocking hierarchies that informed understandings of the epidemic—hierarchies that placed "innocent" PWAs over "guilty" ones, white PWAs over Black and Brown PWAs, and tolerant, educated people over a backward and ignorant "general public." These hierarchies would structure the 1989 made-for-television movie focused on the Ryan White saga.

CHAPTER FOUR

THE "COUNTRY HICKS" OF KOKOMO

The people of Kokomo feel sorry for Ryan White, but they insist on their right to protect their children as they see fit. Many of the parents of Kokomo say that by protecting their children they are being portrayed in the news media as a bunch of ignorant rednecks.

Michael Specter, *Washington Post*, 1985

As Ryan White became "the best known AIDS victim in the United States if not the world" in the latter half of the 1980s, the news media and popular narratives that swirled around him increasingly focused on the importance of education and tolerance within the AIDS epidemic.[1] Just as Ryan's fame and visibility required the marginalization of other people with AIDS—namely queer people, intravenous drug users, and people of color—the emphasis on awareness and acceptance in the Ryan White saga required the countervailing forces of ignorance and intolerance. The communities of Kokomo and Russiaville, where the White family fought valiantly to affirm Ryan's right to attend school, came to represent these forces, especially after the Whites moved to the small town of Cicero, Indiana, in 1987. News media and other popular narratives stressed the fact that Ryan and his family had been embraced by the locals in Cicero and in the neighboring communities, including Arcadia, home to Hamilton Heights High School.

Depictions of Kokomo and Russiaville as ignorant and reactionary assumed familiar class, regional, and spatial dimensions. AIDS erupted at a moment in which racism, sexism, homophobia, and other prejudices were increasingly cast as personal or cultural failures, rather than systemic problems, and a moment in which poor, working-class, and rural whites increasingly became the faces of bigotry in the national imagination.[2] During and after the 1970s, musicologist Nadine Hubbs shows, American society witnessed "a gradual *middle-classing of the queer*," through which "sexual and gender deviance" were "recast, in various ways domesticated, and moved upmarket, brought from working-class disrepute into the respectable realm of the middle class." No longer an acceptable feature of polite middle- or ruling-class society, homophobia increasingly became associated with the poor, the working class, and the undereducated. "Rednecks," "white trash," and "hillbillies," Hubbs writes, emerged in the latter parts of the twentieth century as "the backward, intolerant, guilty party in America's homophobia problem."[3] The popularity of such stereotypes ultimately helped individualize the problem of homophobia while obscuring its structural and material foundations.

"Colorblind" rhetoric, ideology, and culture—ascendant during Ryan White's time in the limelight from 1985 until his death in 1990—operated on similar logics. As Justin Gomer demonstrates in his study of "colorblind cinema," Hollywood treatments of race in the "post–civil rights" era—particularly beginning in the Reagan years—frequently represented "white bigots" as the ultimate purveyors and enactors of racism. In films like *Mississippi Burning* (1988), *Glory* (1989), *The Long Walk Home* (1990), *Ghosts of Mississippi* (1996), and more recently *The Help* (2011), onscreen racists "provide a culprit for the racism the black characters experience" and "serve as a source of blame for past racial sins" in a way "that does not implicate the colorblind hero[es]" of these films. On the contrary, centering the socially unacceptable actions and attitudes of white racists works "to display the heroism of the colorblind [white] protagonist."[4] These movies thereby encourage white audiences to distance themselves from cartoonish white bigots—coded as poor, working class, and undereducated—and to recognize individualized tolerance and "colorblindness" as appropriate solutions to deeply entrenched systems of white supremacy, settler colonialism, and anti-Black racism.

A 1989 made-for-TV movie dramatizing the Ryan White saga exemplified similar themes by individualizing the AIDS crisis and the related problem of homophobia. Broadcast on ABC, *The Ryan White Story* depicts White's struggles for acceptance in Kokomo and his family's eventual escape to Cicero, whose townspeople seemingly welcomed Ryan, his mother, and his sister, Andrea, with open arms. Not unlike "colorblind" films—which understand racism as an affliction suffered by ugly, backward individuals—*The Ryan White Story* casts HIV/AIDS discrimination as a personal problem instead of a symptom of institutional homophobia, racism, and antidrug stigma, processes to which the film arguably contributed by uncritically spotlighting an "innocent" person with AIDS. As *New York Times* film critic John J. O'Connor trenchantly wrote after *The Ryan White Story* first aired, "The vast majority of AIDS patients are homosexuals and drug addicts, but television apparently is not ready to explore these groups with any degree of compassion. Innocent youngsters trapped by circumstances beyond their control provide far easier dramatic hooks for uplift exercises."[5]

The film synthesizes and reinforces many of the themes that coursed through news media coverage of the Ryan White saga. Specifically, it portrays Kokomo and its residents as the main source of White's troubles. The writers and producers of the television movie consulted extensively with the White family, who regularly visited the set in Statesville, North Carolina, during the filming process.[6] Accordingly, the movie largely replicates the narrative articulated by Ryan and Jeanne White, various news media outlets, and many observers within and beyond Kokomo. In this dominant narrative, Kokomoans and the Western School Corporation, which initially barred Ryan from attending school in the area, made life miserable for the White family. Kokomo's deep-seated homophobia and general backwardness ultimately forced the Whites to decamp for the kinder, more welcoming town of Cicero.

This narrative—and the news media and pop cultural products that gave it life—identified personal ignorance and intolerance as the main engines behind the HIV/AIDS epidemic of the eighties and nineties. *The Ryan White Story*, in particular, puts a classist and regionally specific face on this prejudice, locating resistance to Ryan and his illness firmly within Kokomo's poor and working-class white community. Thus, this made-for-TV film and other texts like it advanced the "national pedagogy" on AIDS, which proposed education and kindness as the preferred antidotes to the epidemic while masking the structural forces behind the crisis.[7] By centering a young, white, straight, and very popular person with AIDS—and blaming his plight primarily on his poor and working-class neighbors—*The Ryan White Story* also reinforced the racial, sexual, and class hierarchies at the heart of the AIDS epidemic.

"THAT HORRIBLE TOWN"

Almost as soon as the Ryan White saga began in July 1985, Kokomo-area residents started to express outrage over news media depictions of their community and the seemingly hasty conclusions drawn by outsiders. As the *Washington Post* reported in September 1985, locals complained about "being portrayed in the news media as a bunch of ignorant rednecks."[8] This quotation reflected the racial homogeneity of Kokomo and Russiaville—"rednecks" are, almost by definition, white—and revealed the antagonistic relationship between many locals and the press. "It may seem the whole country is up in arms against you when listening and watching T.V. and the media," an area woman noted in a September 1985 letter to Western School Corporation superintendent J. O. Smith, "but those I have talked and listened to in my place of business and in the community, you have made the right decision, therefore stand by it, no matter what outside pressure thinks or says." According to this local, "the outside world is manipulated by the media in this situation."[9] In a 2011 oral history interview, Western School Board president Dan Carter conveyed a similar, albeit more conspiratorial, message by linking the national news media fixation on Kokomo with an elitist disdain for "flyover country." Officials in the Kokomo area, Carter insisted, "had the very distinct impression that health people, activists, and the whole country were just waiting with bated breath. Somewhere, there [was] going to be that first student with AIDS wanting to go to school. And we had the very distinct impression that they were hoping it would be someplace in 'flyover country,' rather than on the coasts and big population areas where it happened so that they could control how it was portrayed, so that they could set up 'good guys' and 'bad guys.'" That a similar kerfuffle erupted over the fate of a student with AIDS in the New York City public school system in September 1985 lends at least some credence to Carter's suggestion. The news media "knew how they were going to report it when it happened, and everything they reported was consistent with that template," Carter claimed. "It became very clear, very evident early on, even in early August [1985], how it was going to be portrayed, and we said 'okay.' We're resigned to the fact that we're the villains, and we're never going to change that."[10]

The idea of Kokomo as "backward" fit with broader understandings of the "heartland" as a site of horror, prejudice, and ugliness—particularly with respect to race and sexuality—in the late twentieth century.[11] In a March 1986 letter to the *Kokomo Tribune*, for example, a Carrboro, North Carolina, man named David Lohse described himself as "a 22-year resident (and a proud one at that) of the Hoosier State" who now felt ashamed of Indiana due to White's hardships in Kokomo. "I now sit in horror and read of the travesty of injustice being done to Ryan White," Lohse seethed. "What has happened to this young man is horrible." Lohse also illuminated some of the regional dynamics at play in the White saga, explaining that he "moved to the supposedly backward South several years ago" yet now found himself "apologizing for my Hoosier roots." Through this statement, Lohse pushed the stigma of southern exceptionalism and backwardness onto his home state of Indiana, for all intents and purposes a northern state.[12] Similar notions of regional backwardness informed a San Francisco man's letter to the *Kokomo Tribune*. "We in the West," he wrote, "are watching with interest the brutal treatment of Ryan White by the flower of Midwestern parenthood and Christianity. Frankly, after watching the television coverage of the parents' meetings, I can see why corn and swine thrive in America's heartland."[13]

Locals in Kokomo, Russiaville, and the surrounding areas picked up on, and objected to, the classist and regionally specific criticisms leveled against their communities. Kokomo mayor Stephen Daily invited various community leaders "into his office to talk about what we can do to improve the image of Kokomo," local minister Reverend Ruth Lawson recalled in a 2011 oral history interview. "And I can remember that he had a picture that someone had drawn, a cartoon. . . . And it had this billboard, and it looked like the depiction of, like, Tennessee hillbillies . . . with the straw coming out of their mouth and the holes in their hats and the overall[s] and blue jeans." The billboard, Lawson remembered, read something along the lines of, "Welcome to Kokomo, unless you have AIDS." For Lawson, "it was just a real depiction that these are . . . that we were really backwards and had no understanding of life or issues, and we're all just hicks, and just very crude and mean to people. And that was the main focus about Kokomo at that time."[14] In September 1987, after Ryan had moved to Cicero and enrolled at Hamilton Heights High School in Arcadia, Mayor Daily wrote a letter to the editor of the *Fort Wayne News Sentinel* noting that "Arcadia, Ind., too, had its apprehensions" about admitting Ryan White. Yet through state-sponsored education and training, these "apprehensions" melted away, Daily indicated. By contrast, those in Howard County "did not have the advantage of that state-provided education." Rather, they had been inundated with "scare headlines and sensationalist exploitation of a national crisis. On such an information base," Daily wrote, "it is difficult to . . . prune back one's fears through the use of reason." Although some "repugnant" individuals "deserve whatever label is applied," Daily insisted, other locals "do not deserve the portrayal of their community and, therefore, themselves, as a collection of mindless rustics wallowing in their own benighted ignorance."[15]

Some quibbled with the very rationale behind the Whites' move. How could a community located just thirty miles away be so different, so much more tolerant than Kokomo and Russiaville, especially when that community had its own sordid past? In a 2011 oral history interview, Wanda

Bilodeau, sister of Ryan's best friend, Heath Bowen, said that she "thought it was unfortunate on a national level" that Kokomo became "the bad town. 'They hated Ryan. They treated him so poorly.'" Conversely, Cicero was ostensibly chock-full of "nice, sweet, loving people welcoming [Ryan] with open arms."[16] The entire story seemed off. John Wiles, the former editor of the *Kokomo Tribune*, felt the same way. "You know," Wiles asked incredulously in a 2008 oral history interview, "how are you escaping bigotry by moving about twenty miles south in Hamilton County, which was known and [is] still known today as Klan headquarters of Indiana? And yet all [news media accounts] said was, you know, 'bigot-free country.'"[17] As Wiles suggested, Hamilton County—like many parts of Indiana—had been a hotbed of Ku Klux Klan activity in the 1920s.[18]

Despite locals' objections at the time, conceptions of Kokomo as "the bad town" persisted and flourished in the late 1980s, and they would shape *The Ryan White Story*.[19] An August 1988 *NBC Nightly News* story discussed the made-for-TV film and the Whites' role in developing it. Interviewed on the film set in North Carolina, Ryan told a national audience about his hopes for the film. "I hope it shows how we really dealt with it and how, you know, what really went on and how much trouble we really went through."[20] The movie certainly foregrounded such trouble. In so doing, it exemplified and advanced the classist assumptions undergirding not only the White saga but also mainstream discourse pertaining to racism, homophobia, and bigotry in the late twentieth-century United States.

THE RYAN WHITE STORY AND ITS DISCONTENTS

Even before ABC first broadcast *The Ryan White Story* in January 1989, concerns about the film's accuracy and fairness proliferated. Considering the intense and consistent criticism that Kokomo had already endured in the popular press, Stephen Daily and other townspeople dreaded the film's release. "*The Ryan White Story* seems likely to reawaken that bitterness in [Kokomo] residents," the *Indianapolis Star* noted about a month before the movie aired, and when the *Star* offered to preview the film for Daily, he declined. "Nobody is proud of the way Ryan was treated," Daily admitted, "but I think by and large the majority of people in Kokomo reacted very well. You have to remember how little we knew about AIDS at the time." Seemingly resigned to his town's fate, however, Daily declared, "There's no doubt in my mind [the film is] not going to be fair, but quite frankly I'm tired of fighting that battle." He went on to exclaim, "I'm sick to death of what this thing has done to this community." Jeanne White, of course, disagreed with Daily, and although she characterized the film as "excellent," she added, "It doesn't portray them [Kokomo residents] as bad as they really were. They were a lot worse than what the movie shows. . . . The extremes the community went to to keep Ryan out [of school] were just unbelievable."[21]

While public relations figures associated with the film confessed that many locals would find the film's portrayal of Kokomo and Howard County distasteful, they also insisted that the area "won't be treated unfairly." As one ABC spokesman named Jim Butler put it, "It's not [conveyed] like a town of AIDS Ku Klux Klan. Ryan doesn't feel that way." Though he looked to deny any presumed linkage between Kokomo and the KKK, Butler nonetheless injected the violent bigotry so intimately associated with the Klan directly into conversations about Kokomo's mistreatment of a vulnerable boy stricken with a deadly, stigmatized illness. The fact that the town had also seen major Klan activity earlier in the twentieth century could only tighten the association between Kokomo and white bigotry.[22]

Feeding into conceptions of AIDS as primarily a problem of willful ignorance and intolerance, the National Education Association created and distributed a study guide to accompany *The Ryan White Story*. In a memorandum introducing the study guide, the association's president and executive director justified the study guide's focus on education and personal behavior. "Only through understanding," they wrote, "can the fear around AIDS be overcome—and a real start be made toward preventing the behaviors that put young people at risk for this tragic disease." Accordingly, the study guide outlined "classroom activities and resources that our members can use to broaden understanding about AIDS and prejudice."[23] Among other objectives, the study guide sought "to increase awareness about personal, family and community issues related to hemophilia and Acquired Immunodeficiency Syndrome (AIDS) in children," "to understand and evaluate myths that would limit affected students' access to education, peer relationships or community life," and "to impart factual information that will halt the spread of the AIDS virus."[24] The study guide thus advanced the "national pedagogy" on AIDS. Education and tolerance supplied potential antidotes to the epidemic, while ignorance and intolerance—concepts freighted with racial, class, and regional significance—served as its main engines.

Some 15 million Americans tuned in to see the initial broadcast of *The Ryan White Story*, making it the second most-watched television program on the night of Monday, January 16, 1989.[25] The film opens with a montage set to John Cougar Mellencamp's 1985 song "Small Town." Scenes from downtown

Indianapolis appear—touristy sights but also pawnshops, homeless shelters, and other reminders of the abject poverty and suffering in which many urban dwellers lived and continue to live. The movie then takes the viewer on a road trip north to Kokomo, passing highway markers, billboards, and pastoral scenes that reflect Mellencamp's lyrics—"I was born in a small town / And I live in a small town / Probably die in a small town." The montage finally ends in Kokomo, where it emphasizes the quotidian, the mundane, and the quaint—a sign outside a local candy shop, a man in overalls sauntering down the street, a police officer responding to a minor car accident, and finally the Delco Electronics plant at which Ryan's mother, Jeanne White (played by Judith Light), works.[26]

The film's first act grapples with Ryan's hemophilia and his AIDS diagnosis. Jeanne's mother, of all people, provides the first hint of the discrimination and hostility Ryan and his family will face. "Homosexuals started this disease!" she exclaims. Jeanne supplies a swift rebuke, telling her mother, "Don't blame homosexuals. If you want to blame anybody, blame me." After Ryan learns that local school officials have barred him from attending school, viewers encounter the first angry mob depicted in the film. During what appears to be a meeting of concerned parents, one man announces that his daughter helped Ryan with a nosebleed some time ago, and he is now worried that she may have contracted HIV.

Another man attending the meeting, Jake, emerges as the (unwashed) face of the movement to keep Ryan out of school. Jake sports a stained white tank top, which is commonly (and problematically) known as a "wifebeater" due to its association with poor and working-class whites, who are allegedly predisposed to domestic violence. He also wears blue jeans and carries a rag of some sort, both signifiers of his blue-collar identity and possible employment as a mechanic or plumber. Fittingly, perhaps, the actor who portrays Jake in *The Ryan White Story* (Mark Jeffrey Miller) played a racist firebomber in *Mississippi Burning*, released the year before. Based on the 1964 Freedom Summer murders of James Chaney, Andrew Goodman, and Michael Schwerner, *Mississippi Burning* exemplifies many of the core features of "colorblind cinema"—from its depiction of vicious "white bigots" (one of whom is portrayed by Miller), to its celebration of "colorblind white heroism" as the antidote "to explicit white supremacy," to the ambient sense that "white bigotry" is "specific to and trapped in a particular moment in our nation's history" and in a particular section of the country—the South specifically or "rural America" more broadly.[27]

If Jake's wardrobe and mannerisms do not clearly mark him as a "white bigot," his first lines in *The Ryan White Story* surely do. When the official leading the previously mentioned assembly states that HIV/AIDS cannot be transmitted through casual interpersonal contact, Jake pipes up. "Oh yeah? Then why did the cops in Indianapolis wear gloves when they busted that adult bookstore?" Here he clearly connects HIV/AIDS not just to men who have sex with men but specifically to the presumably deviant and promiscuous men who visit seedy bookshops. Jake also seems to support such raids as a way to discipline MSM and to root out HIV/AIDS.

Jake's behavior in the next scene solidifies his position as a key figure in the ugly backlash against Ryan White. Ryan serves as a paperboy for the *Kokomo Tribune*, but his sister, Andrea, and best friend, Heath, fill in whenever he is too ill to perform his duties. On one such occasion, Heath playfully smears Andrea with fake "vampire" blood as she rolls newspapers. Andrea inadvertently transfers the residue onto some of the papers, including one she and Heath deliver to Jake's home. Stained newspaper in hand (but secured in a plastic bag), Jake—clad in a sleeveless shirt—angrily confronts Jeanne at the White residence. He demands another paper, which Jeanne supplies, but he refuses to hand her the "blood"-soaked copy. "I'm keeping it as evidence," he fumes. Before storming out of the White residence, Jake shouts, "Who knows what could happen to me?!" His stern yet anxious declaration bespeaks not just his ignorance but also his fear.

Jake is joined by a cast of unsavory, apparently poor and working-class "white bigots." Dressed again in blue-collar garb—a red T-shirt with rolled-up sleeves, tucked into blue jeans—Jake chats with another white man coded working class across a short chain-link fence. He tells the man of his unpleasant experience on Ryan's paper route. "Ryan's my paperboy!" declares the unnamed man, who wears a blue shirt with cutoff sleeves. "You mean you can get this from a paper?" he asks Jake with a slight drawl. "Nobody knows how you can get it!" Jake replies before imploring the man to sign a petition to bar Ryan from attending Western School Corporation schools. The man complies. A woman, presumably the unnamed man's wife, approaches the fence with a snarling Doberman pinscher by her side. Her hair is unkempt, and she also speaks with a bit of a southern twang. Upon learning that the petition is intended "to keep Ryan White out of school," she eagerly signs it. "I know him," the woman notes with some agitation. "I'll sign it." Within this same montage, two white canvassers, perhaps a married couple, are coded as upper middle class. The woman wears a conservative

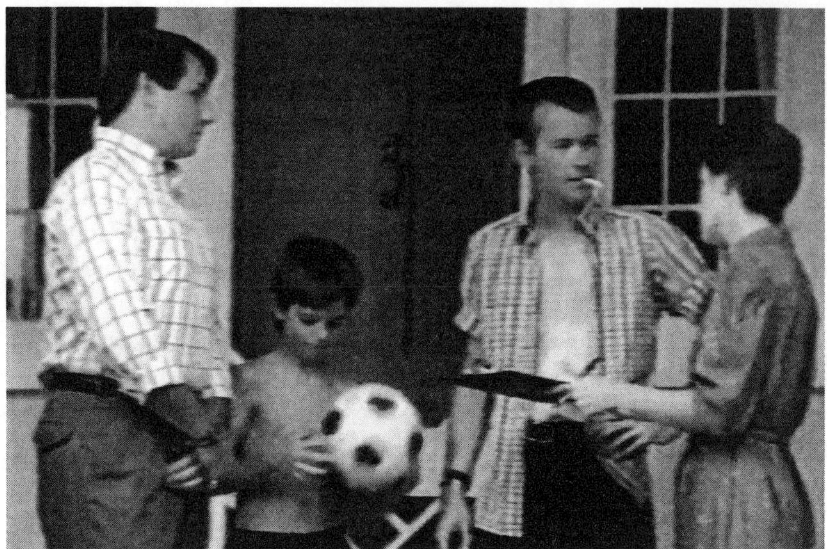

Well-dressed canvassers encourage a young father to sign their petition. *The Ryan White Story*, ABC, 1989.

yet fashionable blue dress, while the man is in a crisp Oxford shirt tucked into blue-gray slacks. They urge another man, clearly presented as working class—a completely unbuttoned shirt, pale chest exposed, lipping on a cigarette—to sign their petition. His young son stands next to him, shirtless, fiddling with a soccer ball. The man agrees and signs. A photographer snaps their picture, which subsequently appears on the front page of the *Kokomo Tribune*.

Homophobia suffuses much of the backlash depicted in the film. On the school bus, for instance, a young girl (speaking with a southern drawl) taunts Ryan's sister, Andrea. "My brother says your brother is a faggot!" In another scene, Ryan tells a television reporter, "People think I'm gay." Locals mock him, Ryan explains, by claiming, "We know how you really got it!"—the implication being that he contracted HIV/AIDS through gay sex. Later on in the film, as Ryan, Andrea, and their mother leave church, two children run past Ryan and yell, "Homo!" and "Queer!" Finally, in a pivotal scene, a teenager knocks on Ryan's bedroom window and shouts, "You faggot!" before running away. Such classed and regionally specific homophobia and backwardness, viewers learn, ultimately inspire a hateful local to fire a bullet through a window of the Whites' house. Ryan, Andrea, and Jeanne return home one evening to find the bullet hole. The film frames this shooting as a clear threat, even though the real-life incident on which this scene is based involved a BB pellet, not a live bullet.[28] "They hate us!" Andrea shouts upon discovering the punctured window. "They hate us here! They're gonna try to kill us next." As Jeanne struggles to console her daughter and coax her into the house, Andrea announces, "This house gives me the creeps, Mom."

This incident, the movie suggests, forces the Whites to move, and Ryan and Andrea rejoice upon learning that their mother has purchased a house in nearby Cicero. Still, Ryan fully expects a chilly welcome at his new school, Hamilton Heights. "Well, here we go again," he sighs as his mother drives him to Hamilton Heights in the film's final scene. "Can't be worse than Kokomo," Jeanne contends. "Yeah, nothing could be worse than Kokomo," her son concurs. Yet Ryan is greeted by a bevy of administrators, teachers, and fellow students, who literally and figuratively embrace him, as Elton John's "I'm Still Standing" plays in the background, and the credits roll.

The town of Kokomo faced tremendous, real-life criticism following ABC's initial broadcast of *The Ryan White Story*. Letters and phone calls condemning the town and Western School Corporation officials poured in from across the country. Many viewers apparently accepted the film's classist assumptions and its emphasis on individual tolerance and kindness as suitable remedies to systemic discrimination. "Ryan is an incredible young man to survive not only AIDS, but the dreaded disease called Kokomo!" Susan Sandberg wrote in a letter to the *Kokomo Tribune* after the film aired. While Sandberg conceded that "this could have happened in any number of towns in Indiana, or any other state for that matter," she noted that "it happened in Kokomo." Accordingly, declared Sandberg, "Kokomo now stands, for all the world to see, as a symbol of bigotry, hatred, narrow-mindedness and ignorance."[29] Responses like this one prompted the city's mayor, Robert Sargent, to write and circulate a lengthy (twenty-six-page) rebuttal to the film. (Sargent had replaced Daily as mayor in 1988.) In his rebuttal, Sargent critiqued what he imagined to be the film's central premise. "When Ryan tried to go to school in Kokomo with the other kids," he wrote flippantly, "the community united in opposition, and in all its red-necked fury, ultimately drove the child and his family out of town."[30]

Other locals found the film's classist and regionally inflected depiction of Kokomo's townspeople particularly "unflattering," as the subheading of one *Indianapolis Star* article put it.[31] Specifically, locals believed that the movie portrayed them as irredeemably backward and ignorant, perhaps to hammer home its message of education and compassion. A resident of Galveston, Indiana, bemoaned the movie's depiction "of Kokomo as an uneducated 'hick town' with unshaven, beer-bellied, greasy-haired men in dirty tee shirts trying to run a sick little boy out of town."[32] Likewise, the community relations officer for Kokomo schools objected to the movie's treatment of Kokomo as "a town of ignorant factory workers."[33] Throughout the film, local resident Amy Royal observed, "the people in Kokomo were portrayed as hicks who didn't know anything. I saw men in dirty clothes, and women in T-shirts and grubby jeans. We were made to look like an ignorant, backwoods hole in the wall town with no knowledge or compassion."[34] For Western Middle School principal Ron Colby, who had advocated on Ryan's behalf, *The Ryan White Story* had set its sights on the wrong villain. "Ryan has an enemy but it is not the people of Kokomo," Colby wrote in a press release. "It is the disease AIDS that was given to him (knowingly or not) by someone else with the disease."[35] Colby's remarks therefore challenged the national pedagogy, which identified uneducated, heartless, and remorseless individuals as the key drivers of the AIDS epidemic.

THE END OF THE STORY?

Time did not necessarily rehabilitate Kokomo's reputation. The residual effects of the White saga and the associated TV movie lingered after Ryan's death in April 1990 and beyond. "Shame, Shame on you! The school & the whole town," Californian Mildred Staples wrote to Colby just days after Ryan passed.[36] In a letter to the *Kokomo Tribune*, an Arizonan named "J. Z." disparaged the town's residents as "heartless, two-faced and still backward and most important of all ignorant." In closing, J. Z. noted that "I feel sorry for your children to have to live with such sickness you teach them. Print that if you dare for all your redneck, backwards idiots and may God help you all."[37] The *Tribune* did not publish this letter, nor did it publish one from an observer in Honeoye Falls, New York, who criticized the "festering philistinism displayed by your homophobic citizenry."[38] In a story that aired on the *CBS Evening News* just after Ryan's death, reporter Frank Currier explained that "Ryan's fight to stay in school prompted a barrage of redneck, backwoods, hick-town labels that still haunt this corn belt community."[39] It stands to reason that *The Ryan White Story*, which had aired just fifteen months prior, shaped such perceptions of Kokomo. Ryan's highly publicized death and funeral in April 1990 only intensified the hatred that so many felt toward the young man's hometown.

Many locals continued to be perturbed by the film—and by its depiction of the townspeople as prejudiced, ignorant "country hicks"—well into the twenty-first century. "I was upset with the portrayal of our community," one of the Whites' Kokomo neighbors, Rita Bagby, detailed in a 2011 oral history interview. "I thought we were portrayed as illiterate, and we certainly looked like we had all dressed like we had come out of a cave or something," Bagby said with a chuckle.[40] Another interviewee complained that "they [the film's screenwriters and producers] portrayed me in the movie as this short, little, dumb hick-a-billy, if you will."[41] In a 2010 oral history, the teacher Cheryl Genovese had hardly changed her opinion on the movie since 1989. "I just felt that they were trying to portray that . . . we were country hicks, and we did not understand what was going on."[42]

The suffering the Whites endured in Kokomo was very real, utterly inhumane, and absolutely heartbreaking. It is also true that many in the greater Kokomo community sympathized with and showed compassion toward the White family. Jeanne's coworkers at the Delco Electronics plant in Kokomo helped cover Ryan's medical expenses, and locals expressed horror and dismay at Ryan's treatment at the hands of their friends and neighbors.[43] Moreover, the hostility, fear, and homophobia that marked Kokomo's response to Ryan White fit within a nationwide antigay panic stoked by the HIV/AIDS epidemic. Two surveys conducted by Gallup in 1987 found that "roughly half of Americans agreed that it was people's own fault if they got AIDS (51%) and that most people with AIDS had only themselves to blame (46%)." Even worse, perhaps, some 43–44 percent of Americans polled "in 1987 and 1988 believed that AIDS might be God's punishment for immoral sexual behavior."[44]

Ryan White's exceptional victimhood—determined by his age, race, sexual orientation, class status, vulnerability, proximity to death, and charm—not only guaranteed him favorable treatment in the press and among the general public but also ensured that those who resisted his return to school would be villainized, as the AIDS crisis was individualized and thus detached from its institutional and structural foundations. In the wake of Ryan's death in April 1990, one Chicagoan expressed his appreciation for Kokomo, because the community "forced us, the public, to take a look at ourselves." He wrote, "If Kokomo didn't exist, and if it never expressed its fear of what Ryan White symbolized, there wouldn't be a Ryan White story to tell."[45] The White saga and *The Ryan White Story*, in particular, reflected a broader late twentieth-century tendency to reckon with injustice on narrow, individualized terms. Functionally and politically similar to "colorblind" films and rhetoric, which co-opted the African American freedom struggle and cast bigoted white hillbillies as the main barrier to racial equality, *The Ryan White Story* and the narrative it presented reduced AIDS to a personal morality tale that stressed the need for education and tolerance—and little else.

CHAPTER FIVE

THE FUNERAL

A funeral in the nation's heartland—appropriate somehow as a place to say "goodbye" to Ryan White, the young man who taught the world that not all AIDS victims are gay, abuse drugs, or live in big cities.

Bob Kur, *NBC Nightly News*, 1990

In late March 1990, several months after his eighteenth birthday, Ryan White fell ill with an "AIDS-related respiratory infection complicated by his hemophilia."[1] He was admitted to Indianapolis's Riley Hospital for Children—where he remained, unconscious and in critical condition, for much of early April. News of Ryan's illness spread far and wide, and well wishes poured in from across the country and around the world. As Ryan clung to life at Riley—and immediately after he passed on April 8, 1990—journalists, elected officials, and everyday Americans alike celebrated the young man as an exceptional person with AIDS.

White's elaborate funeral reinforced his exceptional victimhood. The event was nationally televised and attended by 1,500 people—including dignitaries like First Lady Barbara Bush and Indiana governor Evan Bayh—a far cry from the quiet, poorly attended ceremonies held to honor many other people with AIDS. Some AIDS deaths were hardly marked at all. In his 1987 book, *Policing Desire*, Simon Watney discussed the shameful silence in which his friend's family had been forced to bury their son in a London suburb.[2] Stateside, many funeral home employees simply "refuse[d] to touch" the bodies of those who died of AIDS-related causes.[3] Given the profound stigma attached to the living and lifeless bodies of people with HIV/AIDS, an ACT UP affinity group called The Marys began staging "political funerals" in the early 1990s for those cut down by AIDS.

The responses triggered by Ryan White's highly publicized death and funeral represented a broad range of political sensibilities. But together, they further distinguished Ryan's case from those of other PWAs in the national imagination. The political funerals organized by The Marys starting in 1992 only sharpened this distinction, for these ceremonies reflected the desperation and abjection of virtually every PWA not named Ryan White. While Ryan's funeral had all the trappings of a formal funeral and was legitimated through powerful institutions (the church, the state, and the news media), The Marys' political funerals were fugitive, insurgent actions intended to indict these very institutions for exacerbating the AIDS crisis. At the same time, Ryan's death and funeral helped create the political space in which the federal government would allocate much-needed HIV/AIDS funding via the Ryan White CARE Act. Ryan's demise and the responses to it were fundamentally political, then, and in many ways reflected and reinforced the gaps between "good" and "bad" people with AIDS.

"THE TEENAGER ON THE FRONT LINES"

Ryan's death and funeral in April 1990 were media spectacles long foretold. As soon as White entered the national consciousness in mid-1985, his seeming proximity to death shaped his life story. In August 1985, when Ryan learned that he faced "several months of school conferences and hearings before" the courts would determine whether he could return to school, *NBC Nightly News* reporter Mary Nissenson noted that "Ryan's doctors say he has only two years to live, so several months seem like a very long time to him." White's frequent health scares—marked by lengthy stays at Riley—constantly reminded the public of his vulnerability. As the nurse for the Western School Corporation indicated in a 2011 oral history interview, "Ryan did not attend school much" because he was sick so often.[4] Though Ryan's death had seemed imminent throughout his time in the national and international limelight, he lived far longer than anyone had anticipated, a fact that only added to his legend and broad appeal.[5]

While visiting Southern California in March 1990, Ryan fell gravely ill for the last time. He had attended "a pre-Oscar party" on March 23 ahead of the sixty-second annual Academy Awards, and three days later, in his final public appearance, he joined forces with former president Ronald Reagan to announce the creation of the Ryan White National Program for AIDS Education, an initiative of the organization Athletes and Entertainers for Kids.[6] Ryan reveled in these sorts of activities. According to the *Indianapolis Star*, Jeanne White believed that "her son's hectic schedule is helping prolong his life because it always gives him something to look forward to."[7] Yet Ryan began to feel ill shortly after the Athletes and Entertainers for Kids event. He and his mother promptly returned to Indiana, and soon thereafter, Ryan was hospitalized at Riley in Indianapolis.[8]

News of Ryan's hospitalization and grim prognosis spread quickly. By the afternoon of April 2, Ryan White was "near death," according to the *Los Angeles Times*, and that evening, all of the "Big Three" networks covered the story on their nightly news programs.[9] An Associated Press story published by multiple outlets the following day affirmed that Ryan "was not expected to live much longer," although some close to Ryan reminded the public of the teenager's tenacity and grit. "He's surprised us before," said Carrie Van Dyke, the White family's spokesperson and friend.[10] "We continue to believe he has the opportunity to survive this," Ryan's longtime physician, Dr. Martin Kleiman, noted. "But we have no means to be assured."[11] Ryan was on life support battling a respiratory infection, which *NBC Nightly News*'s Stan Bernard called "the worst infection of his long battle."[12] Although the infection was a complication of Ryan's AIDS, according to Van Dyke, his hemophilia was aggravating his internal bleeding, posing a major challenge to Ryan and the doctors and nurses tending to him.[13] His prospects did not look good.

Anyone familiar with the Ryan White story—from the time it broke in 1985 until Ryan's death in 1990—knew his condition was terminal, and Ryan had come to terms with this fact himself, often waxing philosophical when discussing his mortality. During a March 1988 broadcast of ABC's *Nightline*, for instance, Ted Koppel asked Ryan, "How do you think about the future?" Ryan responded, "Well, I think ahead. You know, I plan my future. I plan to go to college and so forth. But we really live just one day at a time."[14] A May 1988 *People* cover story detailed a similar exchange between Ryan and two students at Father Edward J. Flanagan's Boys Town in Omaha, Nebraska. "Are you afraid of dying?" one of the boys inquired. "No," replied Ryan. "If I were worried about dying, I'd die. I'm not afraid[;] I'm just not ready yet. I want to go to Indiana University." The other asked, "How does it feel knowing you're going to die?" According to the *People* profile, Ryan "shocked" the student by declaring, "Someday you'll die too."[15]

Death had long loomed over Ryan White, then, but with his hospitalization in the spring of 1990 came a general understanding that this was the end. Because few expected Ryan to survive this latest health scare, observers began eulogizing him before he passed on April 8. *USA Today*, for one, published a piece on April 3 titled, "Ryan Inspired Dignity for All AIDS Patients." The use of the past tense in the headline implied that Ryan White's legacy had been sealed and that he would be unable to build on it.[16] The *Chicago Tribune* similarly employed the past tense in a brief obituary published four days before Ryan died. "In his 18 years of life," the piece opened, "Ryan White came to symbolize the tragedy of AIDS. Even more important, the boy from Kokomo, Ind., showed everyone what courage is all about."[17] NBC's April 4 broadcast of the *Nightly News* sounded similar notes (and nodded to the national pedagogy) by explaining that Ryan and his family "served to educate millions that AIDS could not be transmitted by casual contact."[18] Several days before Ryan's death, the TV news magazine *A Current Affair* ran a package that underlined Ryan White's exceptional status in the world of AIDS activism. "Stricken with a disease which claims so many nameless casualties, Ryan was the one we got to know," the narrator declared. Then, speaking over images of Ryan at an Athletes and Entertainers for Kids event, the narrator lamented, "Soon the war against AIDS may lose its ultimate warrior, the teenager on the front lines who battled our ignorance and our lack of compassion."[19]

Ryan's hospitalization even attracted the attention of President George H. W. Bush, who was not known for his compassion or empathy, particularly when it came to AIDS. Bush had just given his first major speech on HIV/AIDS in an effort to shift the administration's tone on the public health crisis. In his remarks, delivered on March 29, 1990, before the National Leadership Coalition on AIDS, Bush proclaimed, "There is only one way to deal with an individual who is sick—with dignity, compassion, care, confidentiality, and without discrimination." Although "Bush's long-awaited remarks" may have represented the "strongest public commitment ever given by the White House to fighting the epidemic," as *Washington Post* reporter Malcolm Gladwell put it, the bar was dreadfully low. AIDS activists were not impressed. Several heckled Bush throughout the speech, accusing the president of dragging his feet and failing to formulate a concrete plan to tackle the crisis. "Why did it take you fourteen months to say this?" shouted one heckler, while Urvashi Vaid of the National Gay and Lesbian Task Force flashed a sign that read, "Talk is cheap. AIDS funding is not."[20] In the wake of this speech, Bush visited Indianapolis, but not to see Ryan. He had traveled there to attend a fundraiser for Senator Dan Coats (R-Indiana), who had assumed Dan Quayle's Senate seat after Quayle became vice president. While in Indianapolis, Bush planted an elm tree to honor Ryan's "courageous battle against a deadly disease and also against ignorance and fear," themes the president had underscored in his address on AIDS the week before in keeping with the national pedagogy.[21]

But the White House had scrapped Bush's planned visit to Ryan's bedside, ostensibly due to the severity of the young man's condition. The decision drew the ire of singer-songwriter (and Hoosier) John Cougar Mellencamp, who spent considerable time with the White family at Riley during Ryan's last days.[22] "Ryan is a symbol of courageousness against [AIDS]," Mellencamp fumed. "Bush was a 10-minute car ride away and couldn't find time. That says a lot for [the] consciousness of this country."[23] While the president looked to soften his image on HIV/AIDS, he had nevertheless refused to meet with perhaps the world's most recognizable and popular PWA in the last days of his life. Earlier that same day, furthermore, Bush had made time to visit a seventeen-year-old gunshot victim in a Cincinnati hospital.[24] In a possible conciliatory move, the White House would send First Lady Barbara Bush to Ryan's funeral the following week. Yet George Bush's failure to visit Ryan—a gesture that would have spoken volumes at the time, given stubborn societal fears of casual transmission and of the "contaminated" AIDS body—could not have inspired confidence in the administration's newfound commitment to fighting AIDS.

Although Bush never made it to Riley, Mellencamp and many other noteworthy figures did, in part because Farm Aid IV was taking place just down the road at the Hoosier Dome. The benefit concert, which was intended to spotlight and alleviate the farm crisis, brought stars like Mellencamp, Kris Kristofferson, and Willie Nelson to Indianapolis—and to Ryan's bedside. Civil rights icon and former Democratic presidential hopeful Reverend Jesse Jackson not only visited Ryan in the hospital but also led the Hoosier Dome in a moment of silence and prayer on Ryan's behalf.[25] Elton John remained at Riley for much of the ordeal, "playing the family receptionist" for the Whites, as John characterized it.[26] "I don't know how I could have managed the week without him, really," Jeanne White later told a national television audience. "That man . . . he shed as many tears over Ryan as I did."[27]

Elton John was so saddled with grief that he nearly blew off his Farm Aid set. Several months prior, he later recalled, he "had happily agreed to join Garth Brooks, Guns N' Roses, Neil Young, Jackson Browne, Willie Nelson, John Mellencamp, and many other amazing performers to put on this show" at the Hoosier Dome. "But at that moment, with Ryan near death, I didn't want to leave his side." Eventually and reluctantly, Elton John left Ryan's bedside to perform before some 45,000 fans on the evening of Saturday, April 7. While the other performers had gotten all gussied up, Elton John "was so upset that [he] didn't care what [he] looked like, and it showed." Clad in a black baseball hat and a red, black, and blue windbreaker, Elton

John stormed through his first two songs, "Daniel" and a truncated version of "I'm Still Standing." He then announced, "This one's for Ryan," before launching into his third and final song, "Candle in the Wind." The arena roared. "The response was overwhelming," Elton John wrote later. "I looked out into the crowd, and people were holding up their lighters, thousands of little vigils flickering in the darkness for my dying friend."[28] As *Indianapolis News* music critic Mike Redmond described the performance, "It was an experience that concertgoers always hope for and rarely get: A moment in which contemporary music's power to grab your heart and rip it out, roots and all, is felt by practically everyone in the concert hall."[29] After his brief but powerful set, Elton John rushed off the stage and back to Riley, where Ryan died overnight.

A DISEASE OR A "DIRTY WORD"?

Just as his hospitalization had been, Ryan's death was a major national story, one that even prompted a statement from President Bush. "All Americans are impressed by his courage, strength, and his ability to continue fighting," Bush asserted, gesturing to Ryan's widespread popularity.[30] In one May 1990 survey, some 88 percent of US adults indicated that they had heard about Ryan White's passing.[31] Because Ryan was so well-known and so well-liked, his death and funeral inspired Americans to discuss the presumed lessons of his story and debate the broader meanings of the AIDS crisis. For most mainstream observers, in keeping with the dominant media narrative, Ryan had personified grace and courage in the face of ignorance and intolerance. The indignities he experienced in the Kokomo area grew out of fear and hatred—forces that were vanquished, first, through Ryan's quiet determination and, second, through aggressive AIDS education efforts undertaken in the Cicero area, where the White family had moved in 1987. The entire country—and, indeed, the world—watched the saga unfold on television and in newspapers and magazines, and Ryan's boyish warmth and kindness helped make AIDS "a disease, not a dirty word."[32] As the Indiana State Board of Health explained just after White's death, "Ryan put a face and a name on the AIDS epidemic. He made the disease real and gave it a human element at a time when most people feared the disease and those who carried it."[33]

However, other tributes to Ryan suggested that his life story and high-profile death had heightened, rather than diminished, anti-AIDS discrimination and widened the gulf between "good" and "bad," "righteous" and "unrighteous" people with AIDS. Since Ryan was deemed an exceptional, innocent victim, many mourners blamed his death on more typical PWAs, especially gay men and people who used intravenous drugs. When the *Indianapolis Star* dedicated its entire "letters to the editor" page to "letters about Ryan White" following the young man's death, three of the fourteen featured letters blamed gay men and drug users for Ryan's illness and ultimate demise. "My prayer," one Indianapolis woman wrote, "is that homosexuals and drug needle users who are responsible for 94 percent of all AIDS cases will accept the responsibility for the terrible grief they bring the innocent victims of their acts—such as Ryan White and his family."[34] Another letter to the *Star* read, "It is perverse to equate Ryan's youthful innocence and basic decency with those who persist in spreading AIDS because of their lust."[35] Clearly, the "human element" that Ryan had supposedly introduced into the AIDS crisis extended only so far.[36]

Building on the popular idea that AIDS could be eradicated through proper education and greater tolerance, others blamed Ryan's suffering, if not his death, on the people of Kokomo. "The harm that your school did will never be forgotten," one New Jersey man wrote to Western Middle School principal Ron Colby the day after Ryan died. "I hope you do something to educate the people of your area of the intolerance shown."[37] In a letter sent several days after Ryan's passing, Chicago public school teacher M. Vic Reiling informed Colby that he used the Ryan White saga to teach his students about acceptance. In his classroom, Western Middle School and Kokomo served "as examples of bigotry and hatred caused by ignorance." According to Reiling, this bigotry and hatred proved fatal. "There is no doubt that the stress you caused this young man contributed to his death," Reiling argued.[38] Shortly after Ryan's death, the longtime director of the *Cleveland Plain Dealer* editorial page, Brent Larkin, penned a piece titled "Kokomo Can Breathe Now, Ryan's Dead." A disgruntled Clevelander mailed a clipping of Larkin's editorial to Colby with the word "SHAME" scrawled across the top in purple pen.[39]

Still others pinned Ryan's suffering and death on the federal government and the nation's for-profit health care system. "White was not so much a victim of AIDS as he was a victim of an inept and corrupt medical establishment," maintained the *New Works News*, an Indianapolis gay and lesbian publication. "If the blood-clotting agent which he was required to take for his hemophilia had been properly screened he would not have gotten the virus in the first place. And were it not for the bureaucratic, foot-dragging, power-playing, fame-seeking, grant-draining and generally stupid medical establishment, a cure would have been found years ago." The *New Works*

News staff also "[found] it ironic that White's last public appearance was with former president Ronald Reagan, who probably did less to promote the end of AIDS than any other living being."[40] A letter to the editor published in the *New Works News* just after Ryan's death similarly targeted the Reagan administration. "More than any other single person Ronald Reagan is responsible for this epidemic. Had Reagan responded responsibly there certainly would have been a blood test much earlier which may well have saved Ryan."[41]

Reagan's obituary for Ryan, published in the *Washington Post* on the day of his funeral, further enraged the former president's critics. "Ryan White touched our lives in a special way," Reagan wrote, and he urged readers to practice kindness and consideration when dealing with all PWAs. "It's the disease that's frightening, not the people who have it," Reagan explained.[42] On a special edition of ABC's *Nightline* that evening, host Ted Koppel called the piece "a very moving tribute" but suspected that it "infuriated" one of his guests, the openly gay *San Francisco Chronicle* journalist and author Randy Shilts, who had spent years covering HIV/AIDS. "It's contemptible hypocrisy for Ronald Reagan to now try to speak moving words about Ryan White," Shilts seethed. "Here you've got somebody who did nothing to help him when he was president now suddenly rallying and talk[ing] about compassion. I think it's absolutely egregious hypocrisy, and Ronald Reagan should be ashamed of himself."[43] For his part, Robert Bray of the National Gay and Lesbian Task Force pointed out the "bitter irony" in Reagan's obituary for Ryan. "His presidential neglect left us a legacy of inaction and shame," Bray told an interviewer. "Ryan White would not have been thrown out of his school if the Reagan administration had called for antidiscrimination legislation."[44] Defying a key recommendation made by his presidential AIDS commission, Reagan had refused, in the final year of his presidency, to bolster federal antidiscrimination protections for those living with HIV or AIDS.[45]

At least one gay pundit defended Reagan's piece in the *Washington Post*, however. *The Advocate*'s Dave Walter admitted that the obituary contained "some incredibly galling remarks." At the same time, Walter wrote, "Reagan also said that there have been too many AIDS deaths and that Americans 'owe it to Ryan to be compassionate, caring, and tolerant toward those with AIDS.'" Walter continued, "As hypocritical as Reagan's words may seem, they just might succeed in prompting a bit more compassion among people who, prior to White's death, did not care much about people with AIDS."[46] This notion that Ryan's death marked a "turning point" in the AIDS crisis proliferated in the days following the young man's demise and funeral. Such framing, which would inform efforts to name the AIDS relief package under consideration in Congress after White, served to reinforce Ryan's status as an exceptional PWA.[47] Indeed, as Walter suggested, Reagan's obituary ostensibly sought to collapse the boundaries between Ryan White and other PWAs, but by calling attention to an exceptional victim known for "his youthful innocence," it failed miserably. "Sadly, Ryan's is not the only life to have been cut short by AIDS," Reagan's obituary read. "In a most poignant way, he told us of a health crisis in our country that has claimed too many victims. There have been too many funerals like his."[48]

"TOO MANY FUNERALS LIKE HIS"

Yet hardly any funerals resembled Ryan's. His funeral service was held on Wednesday, April 11, 1990, in "the gothic expanse of Second Presbyterian Church" in Meridian Hills, an affluent community just north of downtown Indianapolis.[49] Though the Whites did not attend Second Presbyterian, it had been "chosen as the site for the funeral because it is one of the largest churches in the area," wrote Vic Caleca of the *Indianapolis Star*.[50] Some 1,500 mourners attended the funeral, while hundreds more, unable to secure a spot in the sanctuary, were stranded outdoors in the bitter cold and rain. Some, including members of the Ginder family (into which Jeanne White would marry just a few years later), had to be turned away.[51] Many of Ryan's Hamilton Heights classmates attended the ceremony, as did his former foe David Rosselot, who represented the Concerned Citizens and Parents group during Ryan's fight for in-person instruction at Western Middle School.[52]

Unsurprisingly, given Ryan's celebrity status, various stars and dignitaries were in attendance as well. Barbara Bush sat directly behind the White family, and Michael Jackson—one of the most famous people in the world at the time—sat next to Jeanne White.[53] (Jackson had flown to Indiana on Donald Trump's private jet.)[54] Los Angeles Raiders defensive end Howie Long, singer Elton John, and talk show host Phil Donahue served as pallbearers, as did two of Ryan's uncles and his best friend, John Huffman.[55] CNN carried the forty-five-minute ceremony live on air, and all three major broadcast networks showed footage of the service that evening. Ryan lay in an open casket at the front of the sanctuary, his body adorned with some of the clothing and accessories he cherished—and through which he channeled his rock-star idols. A faded jean jacket, worn over "his favorite red shirt," framed Ryan's frail body, while reflective Oakley shades covered his eyes.[56]

A SERVICE

of

WITNESS TO THE RESURRECTION

In Memory of

RYAN WHITE

December 6, 1971 — April 8, 1990

April 11, 1990

2:00 p.m.

Second Presbyterian Church

7700 North Meridian Street

Indianapolis, Indiana

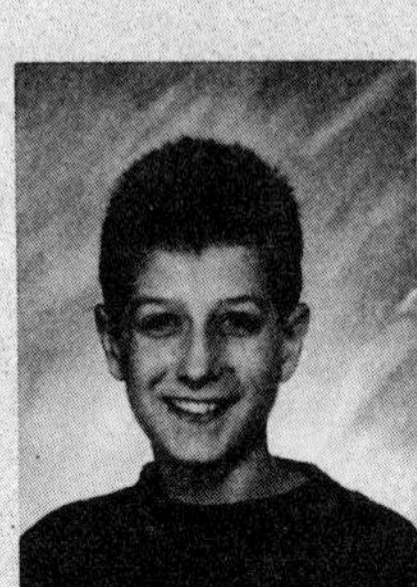

1971 — 1990

". . . I know I'm goin' to a Better Place."

Ryan White

WITNESS TO THE RESURRECTION

Jesus said, "I am the resurrection and the life; he who believes in me, though he die, yet shall he live, and whoever lives and believes in me shall never die."— *Jn. 11:25-26.*

The Prelude

In Quiet Joy — *Dempré*
If Thou But Suffer God to Guide Thee BWV642 — *Bach*
I Call to Thee, Lord Jesus Christ BWV639 — *Bach*
Toccata in E Minor — *Pachelbel*
Prayer Opus 25 — *Boellmann*
Prelude on Hyfrydol — *Swenson*
Cantabile — *Franck*

Choral Introit

His Love Has No Limit — *Bock*
Second Presbyterian Sanctuary Choir

The Call to Worship

Minister: God so loved the world that he gave his only Son, that whoever believes in him should not perish but have eternal life.

People: **Christ also died for sins once for all, the righteous for the unrighteous, that he might bring us to God.**

Minister: God did not spare his own Son but gave him up for us all.

People: **Greater love has no man than this, that a man lay down his life for his friends.**

The Invocation

The Congregational Hymn - The Lord's My Shepherd - *Crimond*
Hymn #104

The Old Testament Readings — *Psalm 27 (Partial)*, *Jeremiah 29:11, 12*

The Anthem

When I Survey The Wonderous Cross — *Martin*
Second Presbyterian Church Choir

The New Testament Readings — *John 14:1-7, 15-17, 27*, *Revelation 21:2-7*

(continued on back)

Special Music

Hamilton Heights High School Choir

The Meditation

The Prayer

The Solo

Skyline Pigeon — *Elton John*

The Benediction

The Choral Response

Go Ye Now In Peace — *Ellers*

The Postlude

Symphony 5 — *Widor*

* * *

THE PARTICIPANTS

Dr. Ray Probasco .... Senior Pastor
Center Chapel United Methodist Church
Elton John .... Soloist/Friend
Mr. Robert J. Shapfer .... Organist/Choirmaster
Second Presbyterian Sanctuary Choir
Hamilton Heights High School Choir

* * *

IN GREATFUL APPRECIATION

The family of Ryan White wishes to express their gratitude to all people everywhere who have supported and assisted Ryan and his family with prayers, thoughts, love and actions.

The program from Ryan White's funeral, April 11, 1990. Bohr/Indy Pride/Gonzales Collection, Indiana Historical Society, Indianapolis.

Presiding over the service was Reverend Ray "Bud" Probasco, onetime associate pastor at St. Luke's Methodist, the Whites' former church in Kokomo.[57] Probasco opened the ceremony with a call to worship based on the oft-quoted Bible verse John 3:16. "God so loved the world that he gave his only Son, that whoever believes in him should not perish but have eternal life," Probasco declared. "Christ also died for sins once for all, the righteous for the unrighteous, that he might bring us to God," attendees responded. "God did not spare his own Son but gave him up for us all," announced Probasco, to which the congregants replied, "Greater love has no man than this, that a man lay down his life for his friends."[58] In this context, observers might have been forgiven for linking Ryan White with Jesus Christ, particularly given the "righteous" versus "unrighteous" binary that had shaped news media coverage and broader understandings of Ryan's saga. Ryan had supposedly died for the sins of others.

Following the invocation and congregational hymn, "The Lord's My Shepherd" (led by Elton John), Probasco shared two readings from the Old Testament, part of Psalm 27 and Jeremiah 29:11–12. The former passage spoke to Ryan's resolve and persistence, even in the face of remarkable adversity. It begins: "The Lord is my light and my salvation—whom shall I fear? The Lord is the stronghold of my life—of whom shall I be afraid?" Probasco likely selected the latter passage to reflect Ryan's sense of purpose and tremendous societal impact, which would be felt long after his death. "'For I know the plans I have for you,' declares the Lord, 'plans to prosper you and not to harm you, plans to give you hope and a future,'" the passage from Jeremiah reads. "'Then you will call on me and come and pray to me, and I will listen to you.'" The Second Presbyterian choir then sang "When I Survey the Wondrous Cross" before Probasco read from John 14 and Revelation 21:2–7, both in the New Testament. In John 14, Jesus consoles his disciples, telling them, "My Father's house has many rooms; if that were not so, would I have told you that I am going there to prepare a place for you? And if I go and prepare a place for you, I will come back and take you to be with me that you also may be where I am. You know the way to the place where I am going." This passage aligned neatly with the Ryan White quotation printed in the funeral program, "I know I'm goin' to a Better Place." The final passage read during the service, from Revelation, discusses "the new Jerusalem, coming down out of heaven from God," and promises "no more death . . . or mourning or crying or pain, for the old order of things has passed away."[59] The Hamilton Heights High School choir then belted out a rendition of "That's What

Friends Are For," a version of which had been released in 1985 to raise money for HIV/AIDS research, prevention, and treatment.[60]

By emphasizing many of the core themes of the Ryan White saga, Probasco's eulogy further distinguished the young man from other PWAS. "It was Ryan who first humanitized [*sic*] the disease called AIDS," Probasco insisted, supplying an alluring soundbite that would be replayed on television news broadcasts and tucked into newspaper stories about the funeral. This idea that Ryan had helped humanize HIV/AIDS not only obscured the suffering of hundreds of thousands of people across the world but also deemed Ryan more "human" than other PWAS—even those (like another "AIDS poster boy," Bobbi Campbell) who hoped to raise awareness about the crisis. As Probasco suggested in his eulogy, Ryan's exceptional victimhood and exceptional "humanity" stemmed in part from his youth and "normality." "He allowed us to see the boy who just wanted more than anything else to be like other children and to be able to go to school," the minister said. "Many of us marvel at the ability of one so young to be able to communicate so articulately the way he felt, thought, and believed." Ultimately, Probasco noted, "Ryan was successful . . . in getting all of us involved" in the struggle against HIV/AIDS. "We saw the boy and the disease, and they were not the same," he added, implying that Ryan's youth and charm had helped to "de-gay" AIDS.[61]

While "emotions ran high throughout the service," Bob Kur indicated on *NBC Nightly News* that evening, the "most poignant" moment came when Elton John performed his 1969 song "Skyline Pigeon" on a grand piano adorned with Ryan's picture.[62] "Turn me loose from your hands," the song begins. "Let me fly to distant lands." The chorus urges the tortured bird referenced in the title to "Fly away . . . towards the dreams you've left so very far behind." Elton John later recalled, "It's a song about freedom and release, and it seemed fitting for Ryan's funeral. Now that he had passed away, I figured that Ryan was free to go wherever he wanted, his soul was free to travel, his spirit was free to inspire people around the world."[63] Ryan's mother, Jeanne, who dabbed away tears with a tissue during the performance, provided a similar interpretation several years later. "The song brought me an image of Ryan's spirit 'turned loose' from his fate, flying 'off to distant lands,'" she noted in her memoir.[64] The memorial service ended with a benediction, choral response ("Go Ye Now in Peace"), and postlude (Charles-Marie Widor's "Symphony for Organ no. 5").[65]

Following the ceremony, Ryan's casket was placed in a hearse and transported, in a motorcade, to the cemetery in Cicero, Indiana, about a forty-five-minute drive at the time.[66] Celebrations of Ryan's life continued along the

KID OF COURAGE
RYAN WHITE
DEC. 6. 1971
APR. 8. 1990
TURN ME LOOSE FROM YOUR HANDS LET ME FLY TO DISTANT LANDS FLY AWAY SKY-LINE PIGEON FLY FROM ALL THE THINGS YOU LEFT SO VERY FAR BEHIND
LOVE
ELTON JOHN
GONNA MAKE IT RIGHT
FRIENDS FOREVER
MICHAEL JACKSON
TOLERANCE FAITH
WISDOM SPIRIT

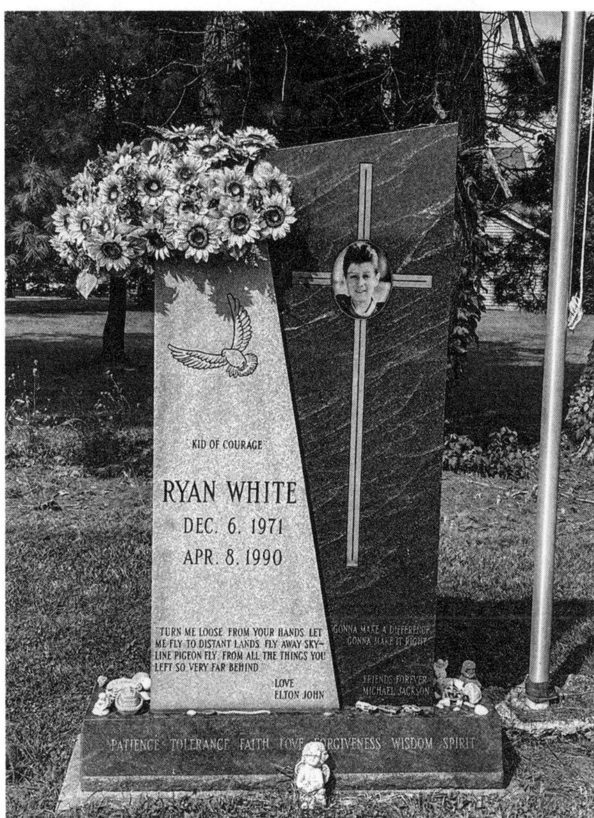

Ryan White's grave marker, Cicero, Indiana. Photograph by the author, September 2, 2022.

way. Many of the flags the motorcade passed would have been at half-mast, in accordance with an order issued by Governor Evan Bayh after Ryan's death.[67] "All along the . . . funeral route to Cicero, on Highway 31," Jeanne White remembered in her memoir, "people were standing, stopped in their vehicles, gathered in crowds at every intersection. Folks stood in front of the fast-food places with their hands over their hearts [and] leaned out of the windows of office buildings and waved good-bye to Ryan." Talk show host Phil Donahue, who rode in the funeral procession, recalled gazing out the car window to see "one of the state troopers who had been assigned to traffic control standing in the middle of the intersection, saluting." That image brought Donahue to tears.[68] Once the motorcade arrived in Cicero, Ryan was buried in the tiny cemetery there, far from the crowds, flashing lights, and glitz that had characterized his memorial ceremony earlier that afternoon.

FROM "SECRET" GRIEF TO POLITICAL FUNERALS

In many ways, though, Ryan White's funeral served as a fitting conclusion to what *USA Today* called a "very public life."[69] Ryan's high-profile life, death, and funeral diverged significantly from the circumstances in which the overwhelming majority of PWAs lived and died. As one Cleveland Clinic immunologist put it in the wake of Ryan's death, "I've taken care of a lot of people over the years who have died in anonymity, hundreds of them who have suffered the slings and arrows of bigotry. No one was there to speak for them."[70] June Osborn, an epidemiologist known for her work on HIV/AIDS, agreed. "We've been terribly short on compassion in response to this epidemic. The atmosphere in America has been so hostile, many thousands of families have had to do their grieving in secret," Osborn told *USA Today* for a story about Ryan's funeral. "There was little secret about the funeral service carried live on the Cable News Network," *USA Today* journalist Debbie Howlett rightly observed.[71]

Ryan's youth, whiteness, perceived innocence, and fame together ensured that his funeral would be a major national—and, indeed, international—event, one that would generate awareness for the fight against AIDS and perhaps garner sympathy for PWAs generally. On *Nightline* just a few hours after Ryan's funeral, former US surgeon general C. Everett Koop claimed that Ryan White's death would help curb anti-AIDS sentiment in the United States. "Until everyone knows someone who died of AIDS," he told host Ted Koppel, "this discrimination and prejudice is going to continue. And I think this winsome little boy has found his way into the hearts of many Americans over the past several weeks, and I think now many Americans know someone who died of AIDS."[72] After attending White's funeral and speaking with some others at Second Presbyterian that day, *Indianapolis Star* columnist Dan Carpenter wrote fondly of Ryan's "countless" friends, many of whom had never actually met the young man. Carpenter highlighted the experiences of Nancy Fleek and her friend Charlene Wiley, who had ridden the bus from their neighborhood on Indianapolis's east side and caught the downtown transfer up north to the "[place] of worship where Ryan White would be sent to his rest." The trek took two hours. In her conversations with Carpenter, Fleek "spoke as if she knew [Ryan] personally, even though she had never met the frail teen-ager with the mirthful features who became an international champion for AIDS patients." Fleek "considers herself his friend," Carpenter wrote, "like thousands of others who knew him only through television, newspapers or letters."[73] These sorts of relationships, as Koop suggested, could only "improve the situation" concerning AIDS in the United States.[74] "Ryan has helped a lot," a "thin and pale" twenty-three-year-old PWA named Philip Hinds told Carpenter at Second Presbyterian that day. "I don't think we'll find someone to carry his torch."[75]

Yet the terms on which Ryan White's funeral generated awareness and sympathy concerned other AIDS activists, PWAs, and commentators. On the day of White's elaborate funeral, ABC's Ted Koppel gently but pointedly critiqued the news media and political focus on "youngsters like Ryan," who served as "safe symbols and thereby deflect[ed] . . . attention from the vast majority of people who have AIDS in this country." While Koppel asserted that "Ryan White and his mother certainly deserve all the support and goodwill that has come their way from the rest of the country over the past few years," he also contended "that the flood of attention which accompanied Ryan White's dying was due, in some part, to the fact that he, unlike most AIDS patients, was neither gay nor an intravenous drug user."[76] In another column for the *Indianapolis Star*—this one published almost a week after Ryan was laid to rest—Dan Carpenter detailed his conversation with a man who had stood "in the gray chill outside Second Presbyterian Church" during Ryan's funeral. The man "was coatless" but "very hot," inveighing against the journalists, star athletes, and pop icons who had secured reserved seats for the service "while people who have stood by Ryan had to stand out in the rain." As Carpenter observed, "The heat of the moment brought to a boil in him [the unnamed, fuming man] some questions that were simmering in the guts of many others who revered Ryan White. 'When have they ever gone to the funeral of a gay person who died of AIDS?' he demanded. 'Where were they in 1981? Where was Barbara Bush in 1981?'" Carpenter agreed with the man. "Ryan White helped make AIDS a mainstream concern by his youth and innocence," wrote Carpenter. "To his everlasting credit, he did not stop there. He struggled, through his debility and pain, to carry the message that 'innocent' and 'guilty' don't belong in the AIDS discussion. Nobody deserves AIDS."[77]

Given the political and media class's apparent lack of interest in the AIDS-related deaths of men who had sex with men and IV drug users—revealed in stark relief by White's funeral—AIDS activists began to theorize, plan, and stage "political funerals" around this time. During an October 1988 ACT UP protest at the Food and Drug Administration building in White Oak, Maryland, artist and activist David Wojnarowicz famously wore a jacket that read,

"IF I DIE OF AIDS, FORGET BURIAL. JUST DROP MY BODY ON THE STEPS OF CONGRESS." Wojnarowicz expanded on this idea in an essay included in his 1991 collection, *Close to the Knives*. Therein he expressed his support for "making the private grief public" through "the ritual of memorials" and recalled "experiencing something akin to rage" during the last memorial he had attended in honor of a fallen PWA. "What made me angry," he noted, "was realizing that the memorial had little reverberation outside the room it was held in." Wojnarowicz subsequently wondered "what it would be like if, each time a lover, friend, or stranger died of this disease, their friends, lovers, or neighbors would take their dead body and drive it in a car a hundred miles to Washington, D.C., and blast through the gates of the White House and come to a screeching halt before the entrance and then dump their lifeless forms on the front steps." For Wojnarowicz, "It would be comforting to see those friends, neighbors, lovers, and strangers mark time and place and history in such a public way."[78]

Wojnarowicz's proposal inspired other activists, including members of the ACT UP affinity group known as The Marys. After witnessing the deaths of several comrades and hearing Wojnarowicz read the above passage during a promotional event for *Close to the Knives*, the newly formed group began to seriously consider the idea of staging political funerals. "We started thinking," member Joy Episalla recalled in a 2003 oral history interview, that Wojnarowicz's proposal "sounds just about right to us." In a 2016 interview, she called it a "Eureka" moment. According to Episalla, members of The Marys gathered in an apartment to compose an advertisement targeting "fellow PWA's who want political funerals."[79] The ad, which urged PWAS to "LEAVE YOUR BODY TO POLITICS," appeared in *Anonymous Queer* (distributed during Pride month) and the August 1992 edition of the *PWA Coalition Newsline*.[80]

When Wojnarowicz died on July 22, 1992, Episalla convinced his partner, Tom Rauffenbart, to hold a political funeral in his honor. Just a week later, Episalla and others—arrayed behind a large black banner that read, "DAVID WOJNAROWICZ 1954–1992 DIED OF AIDS DUE TO GOVERNMENT NEGLECT"—marched from Wojnarowicz's house in Manhattan, down Twelfth Avenue to "Avenue A all the way to Houston Street, up Houston Street to the Bowery which becomes Third Avenue," and into a parking lot, where they held a memorial service. The procession grew to be quite large, Episalla remembered, as bystanders joined the mourners in the streets. In the parking lot at the end of the procession, Wojnarowicz's friends and admirers read passages from *Close to the Knives*, displayed pictures of the deceased, and showcased his artwork. The memorial ended in flames, as participants used the large black banner as kindling for "this kind of bonfire," in Episalla's words. Attendees tossed reproductions of Wojnarowicz's art into the flames in what Episalla described as a "super intense" yet "perfect tribute to David Wojnarowicz." According to Episalla, it was "ironic" that "Wojnarowicz writes this text that many people are [a]ffected by, and he ends up being the first political funeral. It's almost—you couldn't write this stuff. Life is so strange, you know?"[81]

That October, ACT UP conducted the Ashes Action, also billed as a political funeral of sorts. Characterized by activist David Robinson as a "counterpoint" to the AIDS Memorial Quilt, which was on display on the National Mall in Washington, DC, at the time, the Ashes Action enabled activists and allies to deposit the remains of their departed loved ones on the White House lawn. Whereas the quilt functioned as "the acceptable face of AIDS death in the US," theorist and activist Simon Watney contended, it provided little in the way of "social or political explication." For his part, Robinson expressed his admiration for the quilt but bemoaned the fact that "it's like making something beautiful out of the epidemic, and I felt like doing something like this [the Ashes Action] is a way of showing there's nothing beautiful about it. You know, this is what I'm left with. I've got a box full of ashes and bone chips, you know," Robinson noted while holding the remains of his deceased partner, Warren Krause. "There's no beauty in that. And I felt like a statement like this—throwing these on the White House lawn—is like saying, 'This is what George Bush has done, you know. This is what him and Ronald Reagan before him have done.'"[82]

Activists staged additional political funerals in late 1992 and 1993. ACT UP's Mark Lowe Fisher was honored with a political funeral on November 2, 1992, the day before President Bush would lose his bid for reelection. Fisher had left meticulous notes specifying his wishes, which The Marys helped carry out to the letter. After a service celebrating Fisher's life at Judson Memorial Church, just off Washington Square Park, a sea of mourners marched his body—which had been placed in a "very, very simple" casket—all the way to the Republican Party's Manhattan headquarters on Forty-Third Street. As they walked along the route through the steady rain, the mourners held up placards that declared, "MURDERED BY GEORGE BUSH" and chanted, "George Bush, you can't hide / We charge you with genocide." Outside the GOP headquarters, participants gave speeches and paid their final respects to Fisher, after which activists drove Fisher's body in a station wagon to Redden's Funeral Home in the Meatpacking District. According to Episalla, Redden's was "the only funeral home that was willing to do the funeral of a person with AIDS," another example of the different standards by which "unrighteous" PWAs (like Fisher) and "righteous" PWAs (like Ryan White) were treated.[83]

Tim Bailey's political funeral in 1993 further revealed the mismatch between state responses to Ryan's death and those of implicitly guilty PWAs. Bailey had requested to be marched in an open casket from the US Capitol to the White House. On the day of Bailey's political funeral, July 1, 1993, ACT UP members took charter buses from New York City to Washington, while members of The Marys filed into a van, grabbed Bailey's body from a New Jersey funeral home, and made the trip down to DC.[84] When the van arrived at the Capitol, law enforcement officials intercepted it and prohibited activists from removing the coffin. An hours-long standoff ensued, punctuated by clashes between police and mourners. Eventually the cops, including members of the US Park Police and other federal agencies, succeeded in thwarting the political funeral in DC. The incident demonstrated the state's willingness to suppress dissent and displays of grief deemed objectionable—and to do so with force. Whereas police met Bailey's political funeral with violence—thereby preventing activists from confronting the new president, Bill Clinton, at the White House—police had helped facilitate Ryan White's funeral, providing security during the service and traffic control for the motorcade as it made its way to Cicero. Further, Barbara Bush's attendance at White's funeral—and the statements issued by President Bush and former President Reagan to honor the young man after he died—illustrated the state's approval of his activism, the respectable way in which he contracted HIV, and the dignified way in which he was laid to rest.[85]

Although activists continued to orchestrate political funerals throughout the 1990s and into the first decade of the 2000s—ACT UP would hold another Ashes Action in 1996, for example—the decline of most chapters of ACT UP and the rise of protease inhibitors and highly active antiretroviral therapy in the mid-1990s diminished the visibility and impact of these actions.[86] Still, the political funerals of the early 1990s—and the ways in which they were received by political and media elites—testified to the mismatch between the acceptable and "beautiful" tribute (typified by the AIDS Memorial Quilt or White's funeral) and the fugitive, supposedly distasteful memorial (exemplified by political funerals like the Ashes Action or Wojnarowicz's procession). This mismatch evoked the broader distinctions drawn between "righteous" and "unrighteous," "innocent" and "guilty" people with AIDS, distinctions that would define the battle over the Ryan White Comprehensive AIDS Resources Emergency Act following White's death—and, indeed, throughout the 1990s.

CHAPTER SIX

IN RYAN'S NAME

It was called the Ryan White [CARE] Act, cashing in on a child's highly publicized death and focusing on "innocent" AIDS victims—not gays or junkies. . . . No sin, no electoral risk.

Philadelphia Daily News editorial board, 1990

As Ryan fought for his life in Indianapolis in early April 1990, the Senate Committee on Labor and Human Resources—by a unanimous 16–0 vote—reported favorably on S. 2240, an emergency HIV/AIDS relief bill. At that time, the committee members "dedicated the bill to Ryan White and to people with AIDS everywhere."[1] One of the bill's cosponsors, Senator Ted Kennedy (D-Massachusetts), phoned Ryan's mother, Jeanne, following the committee vote. "This one's for you, Ryan," he said.[2] Less than a week later, Ryan was dead.

In the wake of Ryan White's highly publicized death, the US Congress debated the Comprehensive AIDS Resources Emergency (CARE) Act and the merits of naming the bill after Ryan. Religious leaders, HIV/AIDS activists, health care providers, and others weighed in too. While the bill and its dedication generated tremendous support among elected officials, journalists, and the American public, it also drew the ire of antigay conservatives. Senator Jesse Helms (R-North Carolina), among others, downplayed the severity and scale of the HIV/AIDS crisis, thus denying the need for an ambitious relief bill like the CARE Act. Helms and others also considered Ryan White to be an exceptional, "innocent victim"—in more ways than one. Not only had the powerful "homosexual AIDS lobby" supposedly "caused Ryan White's death," social conservatives claimed, but that lobby was now exploiting him to garner sympathy and support for "revolting" practices like gay sex and intravenous drug use.[3] "Ryan White was an innocent victim of these people," Helms asserted, and he was now being used "to promote a political agenda that will put more innocent children at risk."[4]

Some AIDS activists and their allies also expressed ambivalence about the respectability politics that shaped the Ryan White CARE Act, but in the main, gay and lesbian and HIV/AIDS organizations refused to challenge the decision to name the bill after Ryan. On the contrary, they tacitly embraced the move, which had been approved by Ryan's mother, Jeanne. More than anything, the National Organizations Responding to AIDS coalition, convened by the AIDS Action Council several years earlier, remained narrowly focused on ensuring the passage of the CARE Act. And by naming the bill after Ryan, legislators and activists all but guaranteed its passage. Thus, proponents *and* opponents of the CARE Act—and the broader project of HIV/AIDS awareness, prevention, and treatment—sought to instrumentalize Ryan White for their own ends. These developments reveal the power of Ryan's perceived innocence and vulnerability—informed by his whiteness, youth, disability, and diminutive stature and by the way in which he contracted HIV.

The bill's focus on "a politically safe symbol" also reinforced the "hierarchies of victimhood" that defined the HIV/AIDS crisis of the 1980s and 1990s.[5] Once again, Ryan's "innocence" required the "guilt" of already stigmatized populations—namely men who had sex with men and intravenous drug users. While Ryan's "innocence" pushed the federal government to act on AIDS, the "guilt" of marginalized groups fueled the urge "to punish sick people for their alleged lack of moral purity," as one *Philadelphia Daily News* editorial put it. Specifically, the CARE Act contained punitive HIV criminalization and notification statutes and blocked federal funding for needle-exchange programs. Further, Senator Helms's proposed (and narrowly defeated) Ryan White Amendment (Senate amendment no. 1626) would have criminalized blood donation by current or former intravenous drug users and sex workers.[6] The notions of guilt that loomed over the bill also contributed to its funding issues. Though the CARE Act was signed into law in 1990, its grant program would not be fully funded until 1994.

Activists, politicians, news media officials, and others used the CARE Act—before and after it was named for Ryan White—to negotiate the meaning of HIV/AIDS. Before the CARE Act was even dedicated in Ryan's name, the bill's proponents sought to "de-gay" (and therefore destigmatize) AIDS. When the Senate's Labor and Human Resources Committee attached Ryan's name to the CARE Act, the bill's supporters and opponents wrestled over the young man's image and legacy. Whom did Ryan represent? What did his visibility and fame mean for other people living with HIV and AIDS, particularly those who belonged to marginalized groups? These and related questions were debated on the common ground of innocence. In discrete yet overlapping ways, supporters and opponents of increased HIV/AIDS funding both seemed to privilege "exceptional" and "innocent" PWAs like Ryan, a fact that ultimately determined how the CARE Act would be implemented and how the politics of AIDS would develop in the 1990s and beyond.

CHARACTERIZING CARE

Alongside a bevy of other cosponsors from both major political parties, Ted Kennedy introduced the CARE Act (S. 2240) in March 1990. In his remarks upon presenting the bill, Kennedy described HIV/AIDS as a severe and worsening crisis—not unlike a natural or financial disaster—that called for "emergency relief." "In terms of pain, suffering, and cost," the Massachusetts senator noted, "AIDS is a disaster as severe as any earthquake, hurricane, or drought." Kennedy then referenced the recent savings and loan crisis and the October 1989 Loma Prieta earthquake, which famously occurred just before Game 3 of the World Series matchup between the Oakland Athletics and the San Francisco Giants. "America responded within days to the California earthquake," Senator Kennedy indicated. "We have pledged tens of billions to rescue the savings and loan industry. AIDS is a comparable disaster and we need to respond accordingly."[7] Others adopted this framing. "The nation's ability to respond with generosity and support to disasters such as Hurricane Hugo and the San Francisco earthquake provides the spirit upon which this bill [the CARE Act] is based," argued Jean McGuire, chair of the National Organizations Responding to AIDS, in March 1990.[8] As debates over CARE Act funding raged in the fall of 1990, ACT UP circulated a flyer that declared (in all capital letters), "A NATURAL DISASTER IS STORMING THE NATION!" The flyer also gestured to the savings and loan crisis, as Senator Kennedy had, and called AIDS "a catastrophic plague."[9]

Kennedy's remarks in March 1990 worked not only to emphasize the seriousness of the AIDS epidemic and the need for concerted federal action but also to weaken the association between AIDS and presumably deviant populations, particularly gay men and intravenous drug users. This approach, which was followed by essentially every other CARE Act supporter in Congress, exemplified what some critics termed the "de-gaying" of AIDS. In the latter half of the 1980s and into the 1990s, these critics suggested, gay and lesbian groups, AIDS organizations, and their allies increasingly portrayed HIV as "a 'democratic' or 'equal opportunity' virus," not one that primarily or almost exclusively affected MSM.[10]

In one sense, this maneuver accurately reflected the fact that HIV could

A NATURAL DISASTER IS STORMING THE NATION !

On August 18th, finally recognizing the disastrous consequences of the AIDS epidemic, Congress passed into law the Ryan White Care Act of 1990. This bill would at least have provided some desperately needed Federal relief to the cities most devastated by this catastrophic plague. Although both Congress and President Bush have professed strong commitment to this Disaster Relief Program, neither has fulfilled their commitment by finding the funds in this year's budget. Consequently, tens of thousands more will die or become infected needlessly, never having received already promised services.

Congress itself, in its own report "AIDS Treatment and Care: Who Cares?", has said that

> AIDS is a national disaster that can devastate a community as much as an earthquake or a hurricane. AIDS-impacted areas should receive Federal emergency relief funds similar to Federal disaster assistance made available to localities affected by other kinds of disasters.
>
> Within 3 days of the recent San Francisco earthquake, the Federal Government had awarded several billion dollars to the city for disaster assistance. Many billions of dollars have been committed to bail out the savings and loan industry. But no such response to AIDS has been made, even though thousands of human lives have been lost and thousands more will die.
>
> According to the Assistant Secretary of Health, direct patient care services are the lowest priority of any AIDS programs in the Public Health Service, in spite of the overwhelming need for resources to assist overburdened health care systems.
>
> AIDS has exacerbated existing problems of overburdened, understaffed, underfunded hospitals.
>
> The Public Health Service has recommended early intervention treatments to delay the development of AIDS in HIV-infected persons but has developed no plans or program to help pay for it.
>
> The Medicaid Program does not cover many essential services for HIV patients nor does it reimburse for the full cost of care for those services that are covered.
>
> HIV infection is increasing among drug users, their sexual partners, and their children, the majority of whom are black and Hispanic. However, it is persons in these groups who are least likely to have access to health care.

Funding the Ryan White Care Act would not only save lives, it would save taxpayers billions of dollars in health care. The cost of health care for thirteen persons with AIDS currently exceeds $1,000,000. AIDS prevention and education thus makes financial sense. Through early treatment and better case management, people with HIV infection can be kept healthy, avoiding costly and unnecessary medical complications and hospitalization. They can remain in the work force longer and off an already overburdened Medicaid system. Research projections suggest that many could reasonably hope to live until AIDS becomes a chronic manageable disease.

This Act is an opportunity to create and fund community-based programs capable of reaching women, people of color, intravenous drug users and other populations previously ignored by Federal AIDS programs.

In this year's budget, Congress will find the $40,000,000 a day to finance the military presence in the Persian Gulf. They will find the hundreds of billions needed for the Savings and Loan bailout. But they refuse to find <u>any</u> funds for the Ryan White Care Act for the new fiscal year.

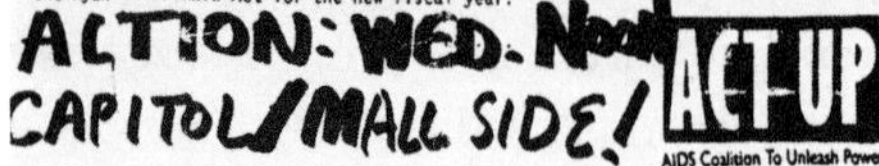

ACT UP
AIDS Coalition To Unleash Power

FUND THE RYAN WHITE CARE ACT NOW !!!

¡UN DESASTRE NATURAL DEVASTA LA NACION !

El 18 de Agosto de 1990, reconociéndo las desastrosas consecuencias de la epidemia del SIDA, el Congreso aprobó la ley 'Ryan White Care Act.' Esta ley debería de proporcionar los fondos federales que se necesitan en el socorro de las ciudades que han sido más devastadas por esta catastrófica plaga. A pesar de que tanto el Congreso como el Presidente Bush han declarado su fuerte compromiso con este Programa de Socorro, no han cumplido sus promesas de asignar fondos en el presente año fiscal. Como consecuencia, decenas de miles de personas morirán o serán infectadas, al no haber recibido los servicios que les habían sido prometidos.

El mismo Congreso, en su propio reporte 'El SIDA, Tratamiento y Cuidado: ¿Quién se preocupa?', ha dicho que:

> EL SIDA es un desastre nacional que puede devastar una comunidad tanto como un hurracán o un terremoto. Aquellas areas afectadas por el SIDA deberán de recibir fondos federales de emergencia similares a aquellos que son puestos a disposición de otras localidades en casos de desastre.
>
> Sólo 3 días despué́s del reciente terremoto de San Francisco, el gobierno federal habia asignado varios millones de dolares a la cuidad como ayuda de socorro. Varios millones de dolares han sido asignados para financiar la crisis de insolvencia de las intituciones de prestamos y ahorros. Pero dicha respuesta no se ha dado con respecto a la crisis del SIDA, a pesar de los miles de vidas que han sido perdidas o que están por perderse.
>
> De acuerdo al Sub-Secretario de la Salud, los servicios de cuidado directo al paciente, no son prioritarios en ningún programa sobre el SIDA dentro del Servicio de Salud Pública, a pesar de la abrumadora falta de recursos para sistemas de cuidados de salud.
>
> El SIDA ha exacerbado deficiencias en el sistema hospitalario, tal como la falta de personal médico calificado, falta de recursos, etc.
>
> El Servicio de Salud Pública ha recomendado tratamientos de intervención temprana para evitar el desarrollo del SIDA en aquellas gentes infectadas con el virus HIV, pero no ha desarrollando planes para su financiamiento.
>
> El programa de Medicaid, no cubre muchos de los servicios esenciales para pacientes HIV+, ni provee el reembolso del costo total de aquellos servicios de atención médica que cubre.
>
> Los usuarios de drogras IV, sus compañera/os sexuales y sus niños, son el grupo con mayor incremento en la infección del virus HIV, la mayor parte de ellos son hispanos o gentes de color; sin embargo, son estos grupos los que tienen menos posibilidades de acceso al sistema de salud pública.

El asignar fondos para la ley 'Ryan White Care Act' no solamente salvará vidas, también ahorrará millones de dolares al sistema de salud pública. Actualmente el costo del cuidado médico de 13 personas con SIDA excede $1,000,000. Los programas de prevención y educación sobre el SIDA son viables financieramente. A través del tratamiento temprano y mejor atención médica a personas HIV+, estas pueden permanecer saludables, evitando costosas complicaciones medicas y gastos hospitalarios. Pueden continuar trabajando y no depender del sistema de Medicaid. Ciertas investigaciones han sugerido que muchos de ellos podrían sobrevivir hasta que el SIDA sea una enfermedad crónica tratable.

La presente ley, es una oportunidad para crear y otorgar fondos a programas comunitarios capaces de atender mujeres, gentes de color, usuarios de drogas IV y otras comunidades antes ignoradas por los programas federales del SIDA.

En el presupuesto federal del presente año, el Congreso deberá de apropiar los 40 millones diarios necesarios para finaciar la crisis del Golfo Pérsico, debe de apropiar los cientos de billones para evitar la bancarota de la industria del Ahorro y Prestamos. Pero se niega a apropiar fondos para la ley 'Ryan White Care Act' para el nuevo año fiscal.

El SIDA no puede esperar un año más....
Estamos ....
EL SIDA NO ESPERA....

ACT UP
AIDS Coalition To Unleash Power

¡DEMANDAMOS LA INMEDIATA APROPIACION DE FONDOS PARA LA LEY 'RYAN WHITE CARE ACT'!

ACT UP flyer in English and Spanish, n.d. [likely fall 1990]. National LGBTQ Task Force Records (1973–2017), Division of Rare and Manuscript Collections, Carl A. Kroch Library, Cornell University, Ithaca, NY.

be transmitted in a variety of ways, not just through anal sex between men. As Celeste Watkins-Hayes has powerfully shown, many straight women such as Dawn Stevens understood this reality all too well. An African American woman from the west side of Chicago, Stevens imagined HIV/AIDS to be "a gay white man's disease" in the mid-1980s. "I was in an all-black community," she told Watkins-Hayes. "It didn't affect us." Then, in 1985, Stevens learned that she had contracted HIV through intravenous drug use. Her diagnosis, Watkins-Hayes demonstrates, belonged within a late twentieth-century "syndemic" that exposed urban communities of color to "overlapping and mutually reinforcing epidemics of drug addiction, violence, and

HIV," all of which derived from "severe health and social disparities." As Stevens put it, "The majority of the people that I hung out with" passed away, many from AIDS-related causes. Yet Stevens survived, saved by what Watkins-Hayes terms "the safety net that AIDS activism built." (The Ryan White CARE Act represented a crucial piece of that safety net.) Stevens now works in AIDS advocacy.[11] HIV/AIDS narratives focusing exclusively, or even primarily, on gay men have served to mask the experiences of countless women living with and dying from HIV/AIDS—not to mention pediatric AIDS cases (a direct product of women with HIV/AIDS), which reached catastrophic levels in New York City and other urban environments in the mid- to late 1980s.[12]

At the same time, efforts to "de-gay" AIDS arguably reinforced dominant hierarchies of victimhood by spotlighting more "sympathetic" or "respectable" subjects. Moreover, this tactic obscured the reality that MSM (particularly in communities of color) *were*, in fact, disproportionately burdened by HIV/AIDS. Many activists on the left disagreed with the "de-gaying" approach, which was embraced not only by Kennedy and other senators representing the "straight" world but also by queer people in AIDS organizations. "It is one thing . . . for organizers to grapple with homophobia and de-gaying from traditional systems and institutions," a National Gay and Lesbian Task Force board member wrote in the spring of 1990, "and quite another to confront it when we come 'home' to our AIDS projects—especially those founded by and based in the gay and lesbian community."[13] For his part, AIDS activist Michael Callen announced in 1989, "If I hear one more time that AIDS is not a gay disease, I shall vomit. AIDS is a gay disease because a lot of gay men get AIDS."[14] As the initial rollout of the CARE Act illustrated, though, many of the bill's proponents would seek to counter understandings of HIV/AIDS as "a gay disease" and thereby circumvent charged debates about its causes—and which populations ought to be blamed for the epidemic. If AIDS functioned like a natural or financial disaster—inasmuch as it could affect all groups equally and inasmuch as it was not "man-made"—then there was no point in assigning blame.

Very few of those involved in the formal legislative process even used the word "gay" when discussing S. 2240 in March 1990. As political scientist Patricia Siplon writes, "Although the gay community contributed enormous levels of support to lobbyists and organizations that pushed Congress to support the [CARE] Act, that involvement would be difficult to discover by listening to the speeches of House and Senate members."[15] Some opted for euphemisms, drawing on the linkage between homosexuality and urban or coastal areas.[16] "The CARE Act recognizes the widespread nature of AIDS," observed Texas senator and 1988 Democratic vice presidential nominee Lloyd Bentsen. "Some think this disease is confined to the east and west coasts. It's true that New York and San Francisco have borne an inordinate share of the burden. But there are AIDS victims everywhere. Texas, for example, has the fourth highest number of reported AIDS cases in the Nation."[17] (Bentsen also used the "natural disaster" metaphor, referring to HIV/AIDS as a "medical hurricane.") By decentering urban environments associated with homosexuality—as well as drug use, crime, and restive Black and Brown populations—Bentsen depicted HIV as an "equal opportunity" virus that threatened not only "deviant" communities but also more "respectable" ones.[18]

Those who did explicitly refer to the gay community sought to loosen the association between homosexuality and HIV/AIDS. While underlining the severity of the crisis, Republican senator and future California governor Pete Wilson echoed earlier press accounts bemoaning the supposed movement of AIDS into the "general population" in the mid-1980s, as if gay men and intravenous drug users were somehow excluded from this category.[19] "We have seen already the tragedy of AIDS spread beyond men of the gay community and intravenous drug users," Wilson said. "To the ranks of suffering victims we now add an increasing number of heterosexuals, women and—most tragically—children." Although Wilson did not explicitly blame MSM and IV drug users for the AIDS crisis, he gestured to the moral and symbolic gap between those groups and straight people, women, and children. Further, he reaffirmed the position of children like Ryan White atop the hierarchies of victimhood and respectability.[20]

The "de-gaying" and de-urbanization of AIDS made the CARE Act more palatable to mainstream audiences, even as the bill chiefly targeted distressed urban areas. The proposed Senate legislation allocated $600 million in emergency relief funding, half of which would go to "the hardest hit top 13 cities in the United States where medical and social systems are in serious peril," in the words of several DC-area liberal religious leaders in a March 1990 memorandum to Senator Kennedy.[21] The other half would be directed toward the twenty states with the largest number of cases "to establish treatment networks in rural areas and smaller towns."[22] Before policymakers attached Ryan White's name to the bill, they took additional steps to make it seem more appealing. Specifically, they recruited other celebrities to generate support for the effort—such as Elizabeth Taylor, who helped introduce the CARE Act in the Senate in March 1990, and *Starsky & Hutch* actor Paul

Michael Glaser, husband of prominent PWA Elizabeth Glaser.[23] Lawmakers also underscored the financial soundness of the CARE Act and its bipartisan base of support, two themes that would have resonated strongly amid neoliberal economic austerity, concerns over "balanced budgets," and demands for "moderation" and bipartisan cooperation.[24]

IN RYAN'S NAME

As Ryan lay dying in Indianapolis's Riley Hospital for Children, the Senate Labor and Human Resources Committee dedicated the CARE Act in his honor. The committee's formal report on S. 2240—published several weeks later, after Ryan's death and funeral—proclaimed that "young Ryan White changed our world." "With dignity, patience and almost unvarying good cheer," the report read, Ryan "introduced to people across America and across the world a face of AIDS that caring human beings could not turn their back upon."[25] The committee report vividly illustrated the power of White's innocence and exceptional victimhood. While "caring human beings" could apparently spurn other PWAs, they could not in good conscience ignore Ryan.

To be sure, the CARE Act was quite popular with legislators even before Ryan's name was attached to the bill. An increasingly visible and militant AIDS movement in the late 1980s and early 1990s had prompted a more robust government response to the epidemic, particularly at the federal level.[26] Upon its introduction in early March 1990, and before it was named for Ryan, S. 2240 boasted one sponsor and twenty-five cosponsors. It secured another six cosponsors in early April. But Ryan's name and image rendered the bill all but unassailable. Calling it the Ryan White CARE Act enabled lawmakers and activists to further "sanitize" HIV/AIDS—and, in so doing, to authorize AIDS funding without incurring the wrath of antigay and antidrug forces. Indeed, attaching Ryan's name to the Senate bill attracted additional cosponsors, thereby establishing a filibuster-proof majority that would keep Senator Helms at bay. By the time the bill passed a (heavily Democratic) Senate in May, sixty-six senators had cosponsored it.[27]

Yet because Ryan was such a potent and popular symbol, the invocation of his name and image by federal lawmakers proved contentious. Everyone wanted to be on Ryan's side. For Ted Kennedy and other supporters of the CARE Act—even activists who may have privately opposed the use of "a politically safe symbol"—that meant passing the bill in Ryan's name.[28] For Jesse Helms and his ilk, that meant "protecting" White and other "innocent victim[s]" from MSM, IV drug users, Hollywood elites, and even certain congresspeople. Through his characteristically cruel and controversial rhetoric, Helms sought to wrest control of Ryan's name and image away from Kennedy and other CARE Act proponents. Although in one sense his efforts failed, given the wide margins by which the Ryan White CARE Act passed, they also revealed the limits of respectability politics in this context. Specifically, Helms correctly identified White as an exceptional PWA who helped direct public attention away from stigmatized groups disproportionately affected by HIV/AIDS, particularly gay men and those who used intravenous drugs. Through this and related observations, Jesse Helms reinforced the perceived symbolic and moral distance between White and other, more "typical" PWAs and successfully promoted policies to further police and subjugate those in the latter category.

As the Senate deliberated the proposed Ryan White CARE Act in mid-May 1990, Helms denounced "the Hollywood and media crowd," the "homosexual segment of the AIDS lobby," congresspeople, and other groups that, he claimed, were "exploit[ing]" White. For Helms, "the cynical exploitation of Ryan White" served "to mask the political movement behind such legislation as we are considering." Ryan's name, Helms told his fellow senators and those paying attention at home, "will be invoked over and over again" by nefarious forces seeking to pass the CARE Act. "The homosexual lobby of America knew the Ryan White story was too good to pass up," charged Helms. "Therefore, his struggle and his death could be used to frighten the American public into believing that AIDS is waiting to happen to everyone, even if they do not engage in illegal and/or immoral activity."[29] Although "little Ryan White was not an IV drug user [or] a promiscuous homosexual," Helms explained, he "was portrayed as a typical victim, not the exception that he was. And the AIDS propaganda machine churned out the demand for special treatment and privileges for the kind of people who caused Ryan White's death."[30] According to Helms, AIDS activists and their allies in the press, the entertainment industry, and Congress strategically concealed "the real tragedy of the death of Ryan White"—that he "would never have contracted AIDS had it not been for the perverted conduct of people who are demanding respectability."[31]

Senator Helms therefore repeated, intensified, and weaponized earlier discussions of AIDS "spreading" from marginalized communities to less stigmatized populations. The "real tragedy" of the Ryan White saga, Helms claimed, was that certain groups had sparked the HIV/AIDS crisis through wicked behaviors and had ultimately condemned innocent, vulnerable people to death. The White story, declared Helms, "told us that children have been the unknowing victims of the madness which brought this disease to Ryan White and America's young people."[32]

Such claims saturated conservative media at the time. In a *Washington Times* editorial published less than a week after Ryan's death, future White House press secretary Tony Snow complained that "Ryan White was turned into a political pawn" and "used to promote an agenda that could endanger innocents like him."[33] That Snow's editorial appears in Jesse Helms's senatorial papers suggests that Helms consulted the piece while crafting his arguments against the CARE Act. In a letter printed in the conservative publication *Human Events* in May 1990, a reader from Spokane pilloried "those who recklessly poisoned the blood supply by their activities, namely the so-called gay community." This letter writer even implicated Elton John in Ryan's death, stating "that his type of sexual union—a prime means of conveying the AIDS virus—led to the very blood Ryan received and died from."[34]

According to Helms and other conservatives, most if not all new HIV infections could be prevented by stamping out "high-risk conduct."[35] Because HIV/AIDS could be eradicated by simply curbing drug use and gay sex, Helms and others reasoned, then there was no need for a relief bill like the CARE Act. In a May 9, 1990, letter to Senator Orrin Hatch (R-Utah), Helms wrote, "If homosexuals and IV drug abusers would stop their disgusting conduct, the AIDS 'emergency' would be over." Helms thereby trivialized the "emergency" that had prompted the Comprehensive AIDS Resources Emergency Act in the first place. In conclusion, Helms explained, "Mrs. White needs to understand that her son died as a result of homosexual irresponsibility—or worse."[36] The CARE Act, funded by taxpayers, would enable such "homosexual irresponsibility," further endangering "innocents" like Ryan White and, indeed, threatening the entire American project. For Helms, the passage of the CARE Act would "feed the appetite of a movement which will not be satisfied until the social fabric of this Nation is irreparably changed."[37]

Even worse, according to Helms and other social conservatives, AIDS was not a serious health concern, despite the claims of the "homosexual lobby" and its powerful allies. For Helms in particular, the "AIDS lobby and its allies in the media" had perpetrated an elaborate hoax on the American public.[38] By hijacking Ryan White's name and image, these groups had convinced Americans that AIDS was a grave, growing, and "democratic" threat—not an isolated one that primarily faced MSM and IV drug users. Furthermore, they had diverted research and treatment funding away from legitimate health concerns, illnesses and afflictions that did not result from presumably immoral behavior. “Despite all of the dire warnings,” Helms indicated, “there has not been an outbreak of AIDS among heterosexuals.” On the contrary, HIV/AIDS had (fortunately, Helms implied) remained localized almost entirely in populations that partook in “high-risk practices.”[39] There was thus no need for Congress to prioritize AIDS funding, especially considering the worthy causes from which AIDS activists were supposedly siphoning resources. Heart disease, cancer, Alzheimer’s, and diabetes afflicted (and killed) far more Americans than did HIV/AIDS, Helms and his colleague Senator Gordon Humphrey (R-New Hampshire) argued, and yet HIV/AIDS received disproportionate attention in Congress, the news media, and beyond. Humphrey, for his part, complained that legislators were “allocating health funds according to which lobbying groups bring the most pressure to bear on Congress.”[40]

Here, Helms and Humphrey were drawing on the work of Michael Fumento, whose book *The Myth of Heterosexual AIDS: How a Tragedy Has Been Distorted by the Media and Partisan Politics* had been published earlier that year. Taking aim at AIDS activists and their confrontational tactics, Fumento argued that HIV/AIDS had hypnotized the nation, directing attention and resources away from more significant and widespread threats to public health. “It is not fair to penalize victims of cancer and other life-threatening illnesses because they do not knit quilts or blockade the Golden Gate Bridge or picket magazines that say things they don’t believe should be allowed in print,” Fumento wrote, lambasting ACT UP and the AIDS Memorial Quilt.[41] “AIDS has prompted a general de-emphasis of other medical problems,” he asserted. “The blunt fact is that people will die of these other diseases because of the overemphasis on AIDS.”[42] Fumento’s claims reverberated in the national press. *Time* magazine, for one, featured Fumento and his book in the January 1990 article “The AIDS Political Machine.”[43] Helms included the article in the *Congressional Record* alongside his testimony opposing the Ryan White CARE Act.[44]

Critics noted that HIV/AIDS was fundamentally different from cancer, heart disease, and the other medical concerns cited by Fumento, Helms, and others. After all, medical professionals had only “discovered” HIV/AIDS about ten years prior, and they knew relatively little about it. Conversely, they knew quite a bit more about other deadly diseases, in part because federal funding for the research and treatment of those illnesses stretched back decades, in some cases. As the bioethicist Timothy F. Murphy wrote in 1991, “Many of the diseases that do now kill people in numbers greater than AIDS have a *long* history of funding, and the expenditures made on behalf of AIDS research and treatment should be measured against that history, not against current annual budget allocations." For Murphy, "an infectious, communicable, lethal disease"—and a fairly new one at that—"ought to receive priority over diseases that can currently be medically managed in a way that permits people to live into old age, a prospect not enjoyed by people with HIV-related disease."[45] In his review of *The Myth of Heterosexual AIDS*, public health scholar Ronald Bayer objected to Fumento's zero-sum understanding of AIDS activism and health care funding. In Fumento's book, Bayer claimed, "those who have struggled desperately to save their own lives as well as their allies' are summarily convicted of murder."[46] Indeed, many members of ACT UP and similar organizations focused not only on HIV/AIDS but on the health care system and the pharmaceutical industry more generally. As historian Jonathan Bell has shown, ACT UP Golden Gate staged a conference in late 1991 that sought to "revolutionize the healthcare delivery system in this country," and the now-ubiquitous slogan "Healthcare is a human right" was first popularized by activist Jim Eigo during a 1988 ACT UP protest at the FDA headquarters.[47]

This capacious understanding of health care justice adopted by many AIDS activists jarred with Helms's vision for medical research and funding. Despite his professed interest in prioritizing the deadliest (and most common) illnesses facing the American public, Helms articulated his support for a more narrowly tailored, morals-tested AIDS bill, one that would benefit people who contracted HIV accidentally rather than through "immoral" conduct. "If you want to consider legislation to help innocent AIDS victims, such as children who have been infected by tainted blood deliberately supplied by homosexuals, we can talk about that," he told Orrin Hatch in the aforementioned letter.[48] In Helms's view, any AIDS legislation named for Ryan White ought to target pediatric AIDS almost exclusively. He objected to the fact that the proposed bill required states to allocate only 15 percent of Title II funds "to provide health and support services to infants, children, women, and families with HIV disease."[49] The senator from North Carolina also expressed outrage at the fact that S. 2240, in its original form, "allow[ed] the States to waive—waive—the money for pediatric programs." He asked his colleagues, "Does that not make the pretense of dedication to Ryan White just a little bit disingenuous?"[50] Yet, by Helms's own admission, cases like White's were extremely rare. "More than 90 percent of [PWAS] caught the disease through illegal, unlawful, immoral conduct," he indicated.[51] Thus, using Helms's own logic, it would make little sense to devote federal funding to a small subset of cases of a relatively insignificant disease.

THE COMMON GROUND OF INNOCENCE

Helms must have known that his cause was futile. An already popular bill, now embellished with the name of the country's most celebrated PWA, would easily pass both houses of Congress. But despite their disagreements over the CARE Act's namesake—and, indeed, over the very need for such a bill—many proponents and opponents of the CARE Act agreed on the primacy of "innocence" in debates over HIV/AIDS. Because Ryan White was such a palatable and powerful symbol, Helms and other conservatives sought to align themselves with the deceased young man—and to position themselves as his protector. The same could be said for supporters of the CARE Act from across the political spectrum.

The conservative Utah senator Orrin Hatch collaborated with Ted Kennedy on the Senate version of the bill and served as one of its most vocal proponents. In his remarks supporting the bill, he underscored (as Helms did in his incendiary testimony) the sort of childhood innocence that Ryan White supposedly embodied. Discussing S. 2240 before the Senate in May 1990, Hatch decentered and absolved those "who have differing lifestyles from others." He therefore refused to "go back to the origination of AIDS and spend a lot of time on that and blame anybody," opting instead for a more inclusive approach that nonetheless spotlighted "innocents" like White. "The least we can do as a Government is help the kids like Ryan White," Hatch said, "babies, unlike Ryan White, who will die before they even reach Ryan White's age . . . help them with this difficult burden and problem of AIDS." Hatch specified "that there are [a reported] 2,200 children in this society who actually have AIDS," although "it is estimated that the number is at least 10 times as great—10 times—or somewhere in the neighborhood of 20,000 to 25,000 children who are infected with AIDS." The Utah senator also drew attention to other individuals at or near the top of the "hierarchy of victimhood" such as Elizabeth Glaser—who, in Hatch's words, "contracted AIDS during a difficult pregnancy." Senator Hatch did mention (by name) the groups most closely associated with HIV/AIDS, namely "homosexuals" and "IV drug abusers." But he advised that policymakers "should not delineate" between the different populations affected. "When we talk about who needs care," Hatch advised, "we talk about children—and this bill takes care of children—it takes care of mothers with AIDS and children, heterosexuals with AIDS and homosexuals with AIDS."[52] While such rhetoric may have seemed universalist, Hatch still foregrounded the "sympathetic" cases that presumably would have resonated with a broad swath of the American public.

Senator Dan Coats, a conservative Republican representing Ryan's home state of Indiana, was even more explicit in his emphasis on "innocence." "Every case of HIV infection is a tragedy, regardless of how contracted," he asserted. "However, the infants, children, families, and certainly many of the women with AIDS are different. They are the innocent victims. They never had a chance. They took no risk and did nothing to invite this calamity. Their suffering is especially poignant."[53] While Coats drew a clear distinction between the "guilty" and "innocent victims" of AIDS, the *New York Times*' Susan Rasky viewed his support for the CARE Act as evidence of "the broad acceptance that [AIDS] funding now has." In a May 1990 article, Rasky argued that "the politics of AIDS has fundamentally shifted in Congress, turning lawmakers who once cringed at voting for money to combat the epidemic or assist its victims into vocal supporters of more Federal aid." Ryan White's death and perceived innocence helped engender this shift, Rasky argued, building on her interviews with congressman and civil rights veteran John Lewis (D-Georgia) and other elected officials. "There is no way we can go around anymore saying this is an issue just affecting the gay community," Lewis affirmed. "In recent days, the life and death of Ryan White brought it home to many, many people." By noting that "AIDS is having a tremendous effect on the black community," Lewis depicted Black Americans and the "gay community" as completely distinct. Further, he suggested that Ryan White enabled him and others to discuss AIDS without referencing homosexuality. "Other lawmakers besides Mr. Lewis cited Ryan White," Rasky observed in her reporting. "The lawmakers mentioned him as a politically safe symbol of the disease's devastation, a symbol that compelled changing the terms of the debate on providing funds to deal with AIDS."[54] Rasky's article appeared to substantiate literary scholar Michael Davidson's claim that "hemophiliacs played (unwittingly in some cases) an important role in securing an image around which [HIV/AIDS] legislation, research, and public policy could be made without having to engage issues of homosexuality and homophobia."[55]

In that vein, longtime Washington, DC, operative Thomas Sheridan attributed the passage of the CARE Act to Ryan White's star power, innocence, and death. As the legislative director for the AIDS Action Council in 1990, Sheridan shaped the CARE Act and helped secure its passage. But despite the popularity of the proposed bill, Sheridan and others had expressed concerns about its "long-term prospects," especially in the face of opposition from Helms and other conservatives. "We needed a superstar," Sheridan wrote later. "And we found him in Ryan White." Ryan's death, which

Sheridan called "both tragic and miraculous," ultimately guaranteed a Senate supermajority that would "break any attempt at a filibuster by Helms." According to Sheridan, proponents of the CARE Act "gained more than just Ryan's bravery, or his sudden celebrity, when he lent his name and spirit to the CARE Act." The inclusion of Ryan's name "helped us circumvent the misinformation, hysteria, and rampant homophobia associated by many with the disease, since most Americans viewed Ryan as an innocent who contracted this deadly illness despite doing nothing wrong. These are not and were not my thoughts, but those prejudices mattered in the politics of the moment." Even though Sheridan "rejected this dichotomy of innocent versus guilty," as did Ryan and Jeanne White, he and other proponents of the CARE Act actually reinforced this dichotomy by centering an "innocent" poster child in their appeals.[56]

The strategic emphasis on a "politically safe" and "innocent" symbol may have ensured the CARE Act's passage, but it also limited the scope and scale of the legislation.[57] The bill, and the rhetoric surrounding it, did not address the structural causes of the AIDS epidemic—homophobia, racism, the unequal for-profit health care and pharmaceutical industries—nor did it fully acknowledge the ways in which the crisis disproportionately affected historically subjugated groups. Rather, the CARE Act's focus on sympathetic "victims" fortified prevailing antigay, antidrug, and racial stigmas, which in turn contributed to the act's funding issues and enabled the adoption (or near-adoption) of punitive amendments during the CARE Act's 1990 passage and 1995–96 reauthorization fight. While Senator Helms's proposed ban on funding for needle-exchange programs and bleach (Senate amendment no. 1624) did not pass in 1990, Senator Kennedy's related amendment prohibiting federal funds for only the former (Senate amendment no. 1625) did.[58] (Kennedy's amendment actually reinforced an existing federal ban on needle- and syringe-exchange programs, which had been introduced by Helms in 1988.)[59] Similar antidrug and antigay exclusions would find their way into the CARE Act reauthorization bill in the mid-1990s.

Efforts to criminalize behaviors that might lead to HIV transmission traced back to the mid-1980s, but the Ryan White CARE Act expanded and formalized such efforts. As Dini Harsono, Carol L. Galletly, Elaine O'Keefe, and Zita Lazzarini have shown, the CARE Act represented "an important milestone in the development of US HIV exposure laws." In order to receive federal funds under the Ryan White CARE Act, states were required to establish and maintain mechanisms through which "to prosecute HIV-infected individuals who knowingly exposed others to HIV."[60] Earlier state and local efforts to criminalize the potential transmission of HIV hinged upon notions of sex-crazed "HIV monsters" indiscriminately infecting "innocents."[61] In the eighties, sociologist Trevor Hoppe writes, many law enforcement officials and policymakers identified sex workers as vectors of disease who threatened the "general population," a category that implicitly excluded gay men and other historically subjugated groups. As these actors saw it, "prostitutes were not just killing their clients[;] they were endangering the lives of innocent women and children."[62] The Ryan White CARE Act, and the criminalization statute tucked within it, intensified and legitimated these sorts of claims—juxtaposing "innocent" PWAs such as Ryan with the less "respectable" intravenous drug users, sex workers, and gay men who were ostensibly driving the HIV/AIDS epidemic. As Hoppe notes, "the logic of criminalizing HIV has been propelled at least in part by homophobia," and the CARE Act reflected this logic.[63]

Of course, the Ryan White CARE Act was still a monumental achievement. Inspired by Ryan White's name, image, and life story, the House and Senate passed their respective bills by decisive margins. After an expedited reconciliation process, the CARE Act was signed into law by George H. W. Bush on August 18, 1990, despite his administration's stated opposition to the "narrow disease-specific approach" taken by the architects of the House bill (H.R. 4785).[64] The final version of the bill authorized $882 million in AIDS funding for fiscal year 1991 and $4.5 billion in federal grants through 1995.[65]

Yet debates over funding would persist well into the 1990s, and the full effects of the CARE Act's draconian antidrug and antigay provisions would become apparent only in the coming years.[66] Further, the CARE Act's devolutionary design, which stressed "local control," ultimately benefited "AIDS groups that had been around the longest[,] the white gay organizations that had responded to the epidemic first."[67] Suffice it to say, then, the foundation on which the CARE Act was built—the common ground of innocence—proved unstable and uneven.

CHAPTER SEVEN

WHOSE CARE?

Scientists agree that the central risk factor for contracting HIV/AIDS is *the number of sexual partners*. The more promiscuous a homosexual is, the greater the homosexual's risk of contracting HIV\AIDS [*sic*] and unintentionally (or intentionally) infecting innocent people like young Ryan White.

Senator Jesse Helms, 1995

Jeanne White didn't want to go to jail. Frustrated by the lack of federal funding for the Ryan White CARE Act and by what she called the Bush administration's "official silence" on AIDS, Jeanne had accepted Larry Kramer's invitation to participate in ACT UP's September 30, 1991, demonstration in Washington, DC. Alongside hundreds of other protesters, Jeanne White marched to the White House behind a sign that read, "120,000 Americans Dead of AIDS. Is This Your National Plan, George?" Many of her fellow demonstrators feigned death in front of the White House—"splash[ing] fake blood all over themselves to symbolize death by AIDS"—before padlocking themselves to the White House fence. As the protest unfolded, an ACT UP member warned Jeanne White, "You'd best get yourself across to the other side of Pennsylvania Avenue right this minute because the cops are coming through here and you're going to end up in jail," Jeanne later recalled. "I must say I was very grateful for that advice," she explained. "No sooner had I taken it than the cops came in and hauled off a lot of folks to the lockup. There were eighty-three arrests."[1]

Although the Ryan White CARE Act had passed both houses of Congress by overwhelming margins in 1990—and President George H. W. Bush had (reluctantly) signed it into law that August—it faced funding issues soon thereafter. During a September 1990 meeting, the Senate Appropriations Subcommittee on Labor, Health, and Human Services opted not to fully fund the bill, appropriating only $110 million, even though Congress had authorized nearly $900 million. This decision came down as Congress and the White House sparred over the federal budget, specifically a deficit reduction proposal that would raise taxes in direct violation of Bush's infamous "read my lips" pledge. This battle over the budget led to a federal government shutdown in early October, the beginning of the new fiscal year.[2] Later that month, with the federal government reopened yet still grappling with a "squeezed budget," a conference committee approved a $221 million AIDS relief package, about half of which represented "new money." The other half "continue[d] programs under way" the previous year, before the passage of the Ryan White CARE Act.[3]

Equipped with Ryan's name and image, the unfulfilled promise of funding embedded in the CARE Act, and the support of Ryan's mother, Jeanne, AIDS activists applied pressure on Congress and the Bush administration—and then on the Clinton administration. From the passage of the CARE Act in 1990 to the funding issues it faced later that year, and from the run-up to the 1992 presidential election through the battles over reauthorizing the CARE Act in 1995, 1996, and beyond, these activists fought to define, and secure full funding for, the bill passed in Ryan White's name.

But despite their best efforts, and despite the strategic placement of Ryan's name on the CARE Act, the law had its limits and its excesses. As politicians stressed the need for austerity and discipline in the realm of social assistance, they failed to fully fund the CARE Act until 1994. And in keeping with the prevailing ethos of devolution and decentralization, they privileged local control in the administration of CARE Act programs—oftentimes empowering entrenched, largely white organizations that were estranged from the communities of color most deeply affected by the epidemic.[4] The criminalization statute tucked within the CARE Act also disproportionately affected communities of color, as did other similarly punitive amendments, such as those prohibiting the use of federal funding for sex education and harm reduction practices like needle-exchange programs.

While certainly more receptive to the demands of AIDS activists than his predecessors had been, President Bill Clinton represented only a slight upgrade with respect to leadership on HIV/AIDS. Although certain elements within the Clinton administration supported syringe-exchange programs, several advisors ultimately convinced the president not to fund such programs with CARE Act dollars.[5] (Shortly after leaving the Oval Office, Clinton expressed regret concerning this decision.)[6] Further, President Clinton often failed to prioritize HIV/AIDS in his rhetoric and policymaking. His seeming lack of interest in the issue was made possible by the growing availability of protease inhibitors and highly active antiretroviral therapy in the mid-1990s, which transformed HIV into a manageable condition for those with access to decent health care. As monumental as they were, though, these medical breakthroughs did not signal the end of HIV and AIDS, despite political commentator Andrew Sullivan's assertions to the contrary.[7] They did, however, contribute to the "general sense that AIDS is over," in Michael Warner's words, even as HIV and AIDS continued to upend countless lives in the United States and beyond.[8] In the years and decades after the passage of the Ryan White CARE Act, triumphalist narratives surrounding the law (and the program it produced) would serve a similar function by implying that, because funding and treatment were now supposedly universally accessible, the threat of HIV and AIDS had more or less subsided—at least for those in the United States.

So although policymakers, activists, and other observers envisioned the Ryan White CARE Act as "a living memorial to a boy who died of AIDS," as ABC anchor Peter Jennings put it, the very nature of that memorial remained uncertain and unsettled in the years immediately following Ryan's death.[9] Contests over the scope, scale, and character of the CARE Act thus represented contests over the meaning of Ryan's life and death—and the lives and deaths of other, less visible PWAS.

"A HOLLOW PROMISE"

Though the US Congress had authorized almost $900 million in funding for the Ryan White CARE Act, a Senate Appropriations subcommittee allocated just a fraction of this total during a September 1990 meeting, prompting outrage among activists, caregivers, and others. Public hospitals, "which end up caring for most AIDS patients, [were] most likely to be hurt," Beth Nissen reported on ABC's *World News Tonight*, as viewers watched footage of a long row of hospital beds. The *World News Tonight* audience then learned from a senior vice president of a New Jersey hospital system that "50, 60 percent of the hospital beds" in some facilities "are occupied by people with AIDS and HIV infection."[10] Up against massive budgetary constraints, AIDS service organizations also lamented the loss of federal funding. As Florida's *Sun Sentinel* reported, groups like the South Florida AIDS Network "thought their white knight would come in the form of a federal bill, dubbed the Ryan White Act after the Indiana schoolboy who died of the disease earlier this year." The South Florida AIDS Network "stood to gain $3.4 million" from the CARE Act in 1990 alone.[11]

Some commentators viewed the subcommittee's decision as an affront to Ryan White's legacy. The AIDS Action Council's Tom Sheridan, who had proven instrumental in getting the CARE Act passed, called the move "disingenuous," suggesting that Congress had harnessed Ryan's popularity for purely symbolic purposes. "Congress believes it got its political kudos for passing the Ryan White bill," Sheridan claimed. "But the truth is that they only did half of a nice thing. This is a hollow promise."[12] In other words, the House and Senate had passed the Ryan White CARE Act by overwhelming margins simply to score political points, rather than to curb the AIDS epidemic. Jeanne White agreed with this assessment. "My family and I were honored when Congress chose to place my son's name on the bill," she said at a news conference held at the US Capitol. "But now the act, with no funding, is at best the symbol of an empty promise."[13]

In the wake of these cuts in the late summer and early fall, activists sprang into action, hoping to compel leaders in Washington to make good on their promises. ACT UP chapters staged demonstrations across the country, from Seattle to Los Angeles to Minneapolis. During these protests, activists demanded the full funding of the CARE Act while calling attention to the skewed priorities of the federal government.[14] "Our demonstrations will . . . be an expression of outrage due to the lack of provision of full funding for AIDS care," ACT UP Seattle member Paul Feldman stated before the protests. Feldman and others pointed to the United States' costly military buildup in the Middle East amid Saddam Hussein's August 1990 invasion of Kuwait. For these activists, the United States' mobilization of troops came at the expense of domestic programs like the CARE Act.[15] (As Penny Von Eschen notes, the Persian Gulf War "squelched hopes" that a post–Cold War "peace dividend"—that is, decreases in defense spending—"would allow investment in domestic social priorities" such as the CARE Act.)[16] "In this year's budget, Congress will find the $40,000,000 a day to finance the military presence in the Persian Gulf," one ACT UP flyer read. "But they refuse to find *any* funds for the Ryan White Care Act for the new fiscal year."[17]

On that score, Feldman encouraged activists to emphasize several "messages of the day" during their October 1990 protests: "(1) We demand full funding; (2) Money for AIDS, not for war; and (3) Stop federal AIDS cuts."[18] In Ryan's name, then, ACT UP members and other activists petitioned for AIDS research, treatment, and funding while striking familiar anti-imperialist notes. Throughout the 1980s—even before ACT UP's founding

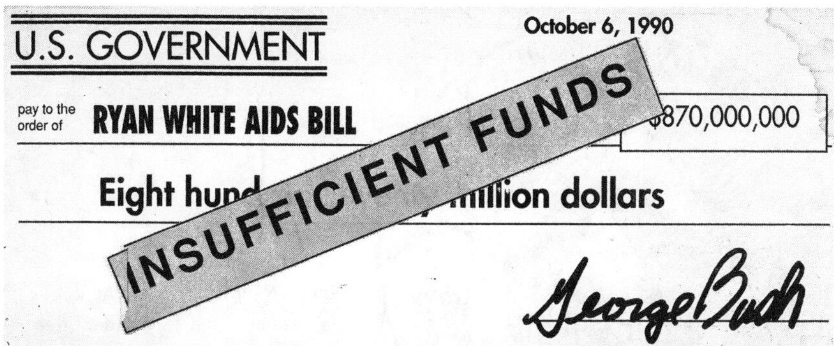

ACT UP / Los Angeles protest sign, fall 1990. ACT UP/Los Angeles picket sign collection (circa 1987–96), ONE National Gay and Lesbian Archives, University of Southern California Libraries, Los Angeles.

in 1987—activists had demanded "Money for AIDS, not war" and "Condoms, not contras," a reference to the anticommunist guerrillas in Nicaragua funded by the Reagan administration. These anti-imperialist sensibilities informed direct-action efforts nationally and transnationally at the time, and they lived on through the advocacy taken in support of the Ryan White CARE Act.[19]

Other, more mainstream actors adopted similar framing, as well. In a *San Francisco Chronicle* editorial that called for greater federal action on AIDS, New York City mayor David Dinkins and San Francisco mayor Art Agnos contrasted President George H. W. Bush's swift and decisive "condemnation of Saddam Hussein" following the invasion of Kuwait "with the glacial US response to another invader that has killed more than 85,000 Americans—the HIV (AIDS) virus. It was six years into the epidemic before President Reagan even mentioned the word AIDS publicly," the pair wrote.[20] Paraphrasing US senator Robert Byrd (D-West Virginia) in a story about the Senate's budget cuts, the *New York Times* indicated that Byrd "objected to the situation, saying that defense programs have increased $756 billion over the past decade while domestic programs increased only $14 billion." As Byrd put it, in his distinctive folksy style, "It's like the runt pig. It's hard for him to get up and stay alive when he's deprived of his fair share."[21]

Protests against the Bush administration continued into 1991, when ACT UP undertook a month-long campaign targeting the president. "The fight against AIDS is not a domestic priority at the White House," read materials publicizing the September 1991 "Target Bush" initiative. "The President has

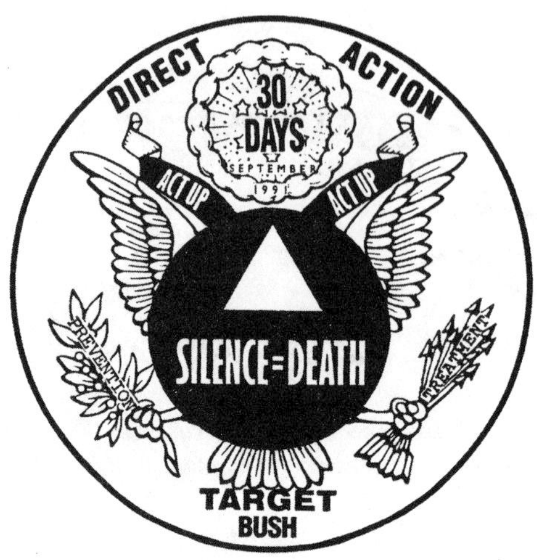

ACT UP New York, "Direct Action: Target Bush," n.d. [1991]. Identifier no. IIP486F10, Digital Library of Nonviolent Resistance, International Institute for Peace, Rutgers University, NJ, https://nonviolence.rutgers.edu/document/IIP486F10.

undermined and undercut funding for the Ryan White CARE legislation." While ACT UP endorsed a more ambitious HIV/AIDS research and treatment program—not to mention a universal health care system—its leaders called for the "full funding of the 'Ryan White Care Act'" as a start.[22] The "month of protests" formally began on September 1, as over 2,000 activists descended upon Kennebunkport, Maine, site of the Bush family's vacation home. Before a march and "die-in"—in which participants carried signs that read "HEALTH CARE CUTS KILL" and "TIME FOR A NATIONAL AIDS PLAN"—demonstrators held a press conference denouncing Bush. They also read Jeanne White's statement written in support of the Kennebunkport action and directly addressed to the president. "If you had lost as many friends to AIDS as I have, you would act up too," White's statement explained. "Please do something, Mr. President. We cannot wait any longer."[23] But despite activists' best efforts, federal lawmakers approved only $221 million in CARE Act funding in the 1991 budget and just shy of $280 million in the 1992 budget.[24]

The gap between promised and actual CARE Act funding became a major issue in the 1992 presidential election. By the early 1990s, gay and lesbian rights organizations such as the Human Rights Campaign Fund had successfully insinuated themselves into mainstream electoral politics—thereby forcing politicians, especially those in the Democratic Party, to at least pay lip service to the demands of gay and lesbian activists. Bill Clinton, then Arkansas's governor, shrewdly recognized the potential power of gay and lesbian voters as he jockeyed for the Democratic nomination for president in 1991 and 1992. Following the advice of a gay friend, political activist David Mixner, Clinton explicitly courted gay and lesbian supporters during the 1991–92 primary season with an emphasis on antidiscrimination measures and tackling HIV/AIDS.[25] Through this approach, the Arkansas governor could distinguish himself from his Democratic opponents, many of whom were less vocal on gay and lesbian issues.

Not everyone welcomed Clinton with open arms, however. AIDS activists confronted Clinton on several occasions on the campaign trail, including during a February 1992 appearance in Sioux Falls, South Dakota, and an April 1992 event in New York City ahead of the New York primary.[26] While the *Gay Community News* commended Clinton for his rapport with AIDS activists and his campaign's engagement with ACT UP, many ACT UP members decried the fact that Clinton "does not discuss his views on the subject [AIDS] at public appearances until prodded by activists."[27] Still, Clinton had apparently done enough to sew up the gay and lesbian vote and secure the Democratic nomination by the spring of 1992. With the nomination in hand, and thus with the support of the Democratic Party establishment, Clinton vowed to "fully fund" the Ryan White CARE Act if elected in November.

In the general election, Clinton squared off against the embattled incumbent, George H. W. Bush. Though few believed Bush could lose the GOP nomination to challenger Pat Buchanan, the prolonged Republican primary exposed the president's weaknesses. The economic downturn of 1990 and 1991 further jeopardized Bush's bid for reelection. According to CBS News polling data, Bush's approval rating sat at a dismal 39 percent in May 1992—just after the Los Angeles uprising and just as the general election cycle kicked into high gear. Meanwhile, 51 percent of respondents disapproved of the president's job performance.[28]

Bush's inability to curtail the spread of HIV/AIDS—or to formulate a compelling, caring message about the epidemic—also opened him up to criticism. By promising to fully fund the Ryan White CARE Act and spotlighting Reagan's and Bush's mismanagement of the AIDS crisis, Clinton sought to draw a clear distinction between his approach to the epidemic and that of his main opponent. At the Democratic National Convention (DNC) in New York City, delegates approved a party platform that read, in part, "We must be united in declaring war on AIDS and HIV disease, implement the recommendations of the National Commission on AIDS and fully fund the Ryan White [CARE] Act; provide targeted and honest prevention campaigns; combat HIV-related discrimination; make drug treatment available for all addicts who seek it; guarantee access to quality care; expand clinical trials for treatments and vaccines; and speed up the FDA drug approval process."[29]

In a direct rebuke to Bush, the 1992 DNC also featured two speakers with AIDS, Elizabeth Glaser and Bob Hattoy. Glaser had found her voice as an activist after contracting HIV through a blood transfusion during childbirth in 1981. As Glaser told those gathered at the DNC in New York, she only learned about her infection several years later, after she had already passed the virus to her daughter through breastfeeding and to her son in utero. In her remarks, Glaser condemned Bush while calling for new leadership in Washington and a new, more compassionate approach to PWAs and to health care, more generally. For Glaser, "this [was] not politics" but rather "a crisis of caring."[30]

Activist and Clinton political advisor Hattoy took a similar tack. "AIDS is a disease of the Reagan-Bush years," he insisted. "We need a president who will take action," Hattoy declared, "a president strong enough to take on the insurance companies that drop people with the HIV virus, a president courageous enough to take on the drug companies who drive AIDS patients into poverty and deny them lifesaving medicine."[31] Clinton mentioned Bush's failures on HIV/AIDS during his DNC acceptance speech, as well. Bush "won't even implement the recommendations of his own commission on AIDS," the Arkansas governor noted, "but I will."[32]

By contrast, President Bush failed to mention the epidemic in his Republican National Convention acceptance speech at the Houston Astrodome the following month. However, the convention did include a speech by artist and activist Mary Fisher, who had acquired HIV from her second husband.[33] Yet Fisher's speech might have been overshadowed, first, by the raucous protests staged by AIDS activists outside of the Astrodome, and second, by Pat Buchanan's incendiary (and profoundly antigay) "war for the soul of America" speech.[34]

Bush occasionally seemed lost on the issue of HIV/AIDS during the 1992 campaign, unable or unwilling to acknowledge the severity of the epidemic and the need for a more robust response. In a May 1992 memorandum sent to his assistant and White House staff secretary, Phil Brady, the president wrote, "The Ryan White CARE Act. Clinton calls for full funding. What does this act do. How much etc etc???"[35] Bush's domestic policy advisor Roger B. Porter replied the same day. "You signed the Ryan White Act on August 18, 1990," Porter told Bush. "This legislation authorizes funds for AIDS-related health care and services."[36] The president's memo, along with Porter's response outlining the basic details of the CARE Act, suggest that Bush was either ignorant or, at the very least, indifferent about the AIDS crisis and the landmark legislation he signed to alleviate it.

In this context, Clinton and the Democrats marshaled Ryan White's name and image to demonstrate that they would handle the HIV/AIDS epidemic with care and concern, unlike their Republican foes. During her speech at the DNC, Elizabeth Glaser proclaimed, "We need a visionary to guide us—to say it wasn't all right for Ryan White to be banned from school because he had AIDS."[37] For Glaser, Bush—and presumably his predecessor Ronald Reagan—had not adequately supported Ryan in his bid to return to school in Russiaville. Clinton, she implied, would have responded to the controversy in a more assertive and more sympathetic manner. In the first presidential debate of 1992—and the only one to touch on AIDS—the incumbent did not utter Ryan White's name or explicitly mention the legislation passed in his honor. His main challenger did. "We need to fully fund the act named for that wonderful boy Ryan White," Clinton announced, "to make sure we're doing everything we can on research and treatment."[38]

AIDS and the Ryan White CARE Act were not necessarily voters' principal concerns, at least according to exit polls revealing a "tide of economic discontent" behind Clinton's victory.[39] But Bush's callous indifference to the HIV/AIDS epidemic surely hurt him electorally, especially among gay and lesbian voters. As Vanessa Williams with the *Philadelphia Inquirer* showed in the week before the election, even Log Cabin Republicans like Philadelphia's Tony Brooks backed Bush's Democratic challenger. "How can any gay person vote for George Bush in '92?" Brooks asked. "It would be just like a Jewish person voting for Hitler in the '30s." For Human Rights Campaign Fund spokesperson Gregory J. King, "There has never been a candidate as good on our issues, including civil rights and AIDS, as Bill Clinton. And there has never been a more disappointing administration than George Bush's." Gay and lesbian activists and voters, Williams wrote, "point to Clinton's promises to end discrimination against gays and lesbians in federal employment and the military. They also applaud Clinton's pledge to appoint an AIDS czar and to fully fund the Ryan White CARE Act, which would provide more than $800 million to more than two dozen cities."[40]

For many LGBTQ+ people, people of color, and other communities disproportionately affected by the AIDS epidemic, then, Clinton's victory represented a possible turning point in the country's AIDS policy, a potential shift in priorities. But issues related to the funding and administration of the Ryan White CARE Act would persist through Clinton's presidency. Simultaneously, the increasing availability of protease inhibitors and highly active antiretroviral therapy in the mid- to late 1990s compelled some commentators to celebrate the "end" of the AIDS epidemic, even as tens of thousands continued to die annually from AIDS-related causes, and even as politicians failed to fulfill the promises embedded within the CARE Act.

DON'T STOP

In an article published to coincide with Clinton's inauguration in January 1993, the gay and lesbian magazine *The Advocate* celebrated "Washington's new attitude." "When Bill Clinton and Al Gore take office Jan. 20," the piece began, "many gays and lesbians will be among those cheering the loudest." Indeed, after twelve long years "of Republican neglect and attacks from the right wing," there seemed to be cause for hope, particularly when it came to AIDS.[41]

On January 1, 1993, the CDC formally expanded its surveillance case definition of AIDS to include women, people who used intravenous drugs, and other previously excluded populations. The decision followed years of advocacy by the Women's Caucus of ACT UP and other groups. For its part, Gran Fury had produced and distributed striking posters and other materials to raise awareness about the impact of HIV/AIDS on women. One 1988 poster featured an erect penis alongside text that declared, "SEXISM REARS ITS UNPROTECTED HEAD" and "AIDS KILLS WOMEN."[42] Another Gran Fury poster superimposed its unsettling message—"WOMEN DON'T GET AIDS. THEY JUST DIE FROM IT"—over a photograph of female contestants participating in a national beauty pageant. When viewers leaned in to read the fine print, they learned that "65% of HIV positive women get sick and die from chronic infections that don't fit the Centers for Disease Control's definition of AIDS. Without that recognition women are denied access to what little healthcare exists. The CDC must expand the definition of AIDS."[43] After the CDC finally changed its case definition in early 1993, the official number of Americans with AIDS increased dramatically overnight, although this revised figure was still probably an extreme undercount.[44] Nonetheless, not only would this new definition make previously excluded populations eligible for HIV/AIDS-specific public assistance and care, but activists also hoped it would spur more investment in research, prevention, and treatment.[45] When January 20 rolled around, Jeanne White and others marched in the inaugural parade while carrying patches from the AIDS Memorial Quilt.[46] Together, these and other developments suggested that the Clinton years would be different from the Reagan and Bush years, especially when it came to HIV/AIDS and gay and lesbian rights.

But Clinton faced both a daunting "full agenda on AIDS," as the *Chicago Tribune* characterized it, and desperate AIDS activists, many of whom were withering away and many of whom had watched their friends die agonizing, painful deaths.[47] As AIDS activist Jeff Levy noted on National Public Radio's *All Things Considered* in the wake of Clinton's inauguration, "If people think that, because Bill Clinton is President, we're going to have a cure in six months, that's unrealistic," he admitted. "But I think it is legitimate for the community to be saying to Bill Clinton, 'You've promised a dramatic break with the past, and if that break does not come quickly, given the extreme nature of this crisis, people will be legitimately disappointed and angry.'"[48] On the bright side, during his first two years in office, Clinton managed to boost Ryan White CARE Act funding by over 80 percent and AIDS research funding by 25 percent.[49]

Yet his failures triggered the very disappointment and anger that Levy had foreshadowed. Activists soon castigated the president for his inaction on HIV/AIDS. For example, a heckler accosted Clinton during a 1993 World AIDS Day address at Georgetown University Hospital. "If you're so concerned about AIDS, where's the Manhattan Project on AIDS that you promised during your campaign?" the man shouted. "Me and my community are dying in ever-increasing numbers, and all you do is talk." For his part, ACT UP cofounder Larry Kramer asserted in 1993, "Clinton is a wuss."[50] Activists had even more reason to be disappointed and angry in 1994. That summer, the president's first AIDS czar, Kristine M. Gebbie, resigned in frustration after serving in that position for less than one year. (The *New Republic* called her "a second-rate hack in a second-rate office.")[51] Moreover, the administration's attempt at health care reform, spearheaded by First Lady and future US senator and presidential nominee Hillary Clinton, died an undignified death in September 1994. As the executive director of the AIDS Action Council noted, the Clinton health plan would have helped tackle "a range of healthcare issues facing people living with HIV/AIDS, from the elimination of pre-existing condition exclusions to the preservation and enhancement of Ryan White CARE Act programs."[52] Nevertheless, the plan faltered just before the disastrous midterm elections in which Republicans seized control of the House for the first time in over four decades.

With the GOP now in power in both chambers of Congress, the prospects for AIDS funding looked bleak. However, the Ryan White CARE Act still enjoyed considerable bipartisan support, perhaps because of the nearly unassailable name and image attached to it. Even the new Speaker of the House, the conservative firebrand Newt Gingrich (R-Georgia), backed the five-year reauthorization of the CARE Act, which was set to expire in September 1995.[53] The Ryan White CARE Reauthorization Act was introduced in March 1995 and sailed through the Senate's Committee on Labor and Human Resources.[54] "Ryan White would be proud of what has happened in his name," Senator Ted Kennedy declared upon introducing the reauthorization bill.[55]

But Senator Jesse Helms disagreed wholeheartedly. In fact, he hoped to derail the whole thing, just as he had looked to block the CARE Act's passage in 1990. Although the bill's sixty-plus cosponsors made it filibuster-proof, Helms managed to "put . . . the brakes" on the reauthorization process, as the *New York Times* put it, because of "the latitude any single member of the Senate has to tie up proceedings."[56] Some observers also speculated that Senate majority leader Bob Dole (R-Kansas) was indulging Helms, refusing to move the CARE Act reauthorization forward in order to shore up right-wing support as he pursued the 1996 GOP presidential nomination.[57] (Dole had announced his candidacy for president in April 1995.)

Helms justified his opposition to the reauthorization by telling the *New York Times* in early July 1995 that HIV and AIDS resulted from "deliberate, disgusting, revolting conduct." "We've got to have some common sense about a disease transmitted by people deliberately engaging in unnatural acts," Helms said in an interview with the *Times*.[58] The angry responses prompted by Helms's remarks revealed the power of "innocence" in HIV/AIDS discourse during this period, as both proponents and opponents of the reauthorization bill sought to align themselves with Ryan White and other presumably innocent people with HIV and AIDS. "It was disheartening to read of Jesse Helms's views of the victims of AIDS and his efforts to cut funding for the Ryan White Care Act of 1990," one pediatrician wrote in a letter to the *Times*. "As medical director of a clinic for HIV-positive children funded by the Ryan White Care Act, I see daily the positive impact these funds have on the lives of children with HIV/AIDS." While this pediatrician observed that "no one asks to be infected with the virus that causes AIDS," she explicitly referenced only "innocent" populations—namely children and "the mothers of the children in my program [who] were infected unknowingly through heterosexual sex."[59] For its part, the *Tallahassee Democrat*'s editorial board conjectured that Helms had "never heard of Ryan White or Elizabeth Glaser, both of whom contracted the disease through blood transfusions."[60] Similarly, one Staten Island man asked in a letter to the *New York Times*, "Does the Senator not know that Ryan White contracted AIDS through a blood transfusion, as did [tennis star] Arthur Ashe?"[61]

Helms most certainly did. Armed with that knowledge, he sought to distinguish Ryan from other, presumably guilty people with HIV/AIDS, just as he had during debates about the original CARE Act in 1990. The "homosexual activists of America," Helms declared in a July 1995 statement, had "managed to convince the news media, and a surprising number of Senators, that it is irrelevant to talk about who and what really caused the death of Ryan White . . . the 18-year-old hemophiliac who died of AIDS because tainted blood was pumped into his veins, blood that was tainted in the first place by a homosexual conduct [*sic*] somewhere generations back."[62] In another statement, Helms explained, "The Ryan White CARE Act was named in memory of an absolutely innocent hemophiliac who contracted AIDS when given a tainted blood transfusion. Of course, I have no quarrel with the Ryan Whites of the world." But, Helms affirmed, "the homosexual lobby has gone to incredible extremes to exploit Ryan White's name in an attempt to acquire what appears to be unworkable portions of federal funding for AIDS, which is transmitted largely by irresponsible and degrading personal activities." Considering that "Ryan White and others like him are a small sliver of the AIDS population"—and that HIV/AIDS "is preventable and so many [diseases] are not"—Helms contended "that we are spending enough money on HIV/AIDS."[63]

Because Helms was blocking the passage of a wildly popular piece of legislation, he had leverage, and he intended to use it. Helms and his advisors therefore strategized over "possible amendments" to the CARE Act, and Helms ultimately introduced five such amendments in July 1995 (Senate amendments nos. 1853, 1854, 1855, 1856, and 1857).[64] Two of these amendments dealt with budgetary concerns (nos. 1855 and 1857), one pertained to spousal notification protocols in the event of a positive HIV test (no. 1853), and another one sought to make HIV/AIDS training programs optional for federal employees (no. 1856). Senate amendment no. 1854—building on existing bans that had been on the books since the late 1980s—stipulated, "No funds authorized to be appropriated under this Act may be used to promote or encourage, directly or indirectly, homosexuality, or intravenous drug use."[65] This amendment passed the Senate by a vote of 54–45, though its explicitly antigay message was softened by a corresponding amendment (no. 1858) proposed by Senators Nancy Kassebaum (R-Kansas) and Pete Domenici (R–New Mexico) and subsequently adopted in the final version of the bill. The text of Senate amendment no. 1858 read, "None of the funds authorized under this title shall be used to fund AIDS programs, or to develop materials, designed to promote or encourage, directly, intravenous drug use or sexual activity, whether homosexual or heterosexual." By marking certain behaviors and populations as deviant, Senate amendment no. 1854—and its watered-down companion, Senate amendment no. 1858—reflected and reinforced the AIDS epidemic's "hierarchy of victimhood" and revealed the limits of the respectability politics enabled by the Ryan White story.[66]

Despite its support for certain HIV/AIDS prevention, research, and treatment measures, the Clinton administration ultimately backed the ban on federal funding for needle- and syringe-exchange programs, a ban legitimated through Ryan White's name and image. The administration's position, which ignored a significant body of research illustrating the need for (and effectiveness of) such programs, drew the ire of activists and organizers. In the mid- to late 1990s, ACT UP New York organized multiple demonstrations targeting Clinton and his opposition to needle-exchange programs—including a "zap" held outside the White House Conference on AIDS in December 1995 and the interruption of the president's speech at a November 1997 Human Rights Campaign event.[67] In 1998, Donna Shalala, Clinton's secretary of Health and Human Services, announced that the benefits of such programs were undeniable. "There was no question that the science was clear," she later told *The Atlantic*. But Clinton did not rescind the ban on federal funding. "The president decided not to do it for political reasons," Shalala noted, alluding to firmly entrenched antidrug stigmas and the stubborn, mistaken belief that needle-exchange programs encourage intravenous drug use.[68]

THE ENDS OF AIDS

After some additional delays, the reauthorization of the Ryan White CARE Act was finalized in 1996, the same year in which the widespread adoption of protease inhibitors and highly active antiretroviral therapy caused some commentators to prematurely declare the "end" of AIDS. Andrew Sullivan, for one, acknowledged in November 1996 that "many Americans—especially blacks and Latinos—will still die" of AIDS-related causes while nevertheless celebrating the fact that the epidemic had entered a new, less-fatal phase.[69] As scholar and theorist Michael Warner lamented in 1999, Clinton's "cynical" opposition to needle-exchange programs "has been made easier by the general sense that AIDS is over."[70]

Accordingly, the president's rhetoric on HIV/AIDS became increasingly triumphalist near the end of his second term. When he reauthorized the Ryan White CARE Act once again in 2000, Clinton placed the reauthorization within a linear narrative of progress on AIDS. Unsurprisingly, Ryan White—and the law and program inscribed with his name—sat at the heart of this narrative. "When the CARE Act was originally created, we were sadly unable to do much for those who were sick," President Clinton recalled. "Thankfully, much has changed. The CARE Act is now solidly about *living* with HIV and AIDS. Since its last reauthorization [in 1996], biomedical research has brought hope and renewed optimism with the discovery of protease inhibitors and combination therapies. The CARE Act has made the promise of biomedical research a reality in the lives of people living with HIV and AIDS in every corner of this country." For the outgoing president, "Ryan White changed the world, and so has the program that bears his name."[71]

On one hand, the biomedical developments of the mid- to late 1990s did make HIV/AIDS more manageable and less deadly for those with access to care. On the other, despite the claims made by Clinton, Sullivan, and others, these developments did little to challenge the antigay and antidrug stigmas that swirled around HIV and AIDS. In fact, the rhetoric surrounding such biomedical advances, which implied the "pastness of AIDS," may have actually enhanced these stigmas.[72] With the advent of new medicines and the widespread embrace of certain forms of medical knowledge about HIV/AIDS—alongside the growing tendency to imagine HIV/AIDS as an "African" problem, not a "Western" one—now there was simply no excuse for acquiring HIV or dying from AIDS in the United States.

Since the emergence of protease inhibitors, the growing availability of highly active antiretroviral therapy, and the globalization of AIDS, the Ryan White story has similarly served to remind the public of the stigma and shame that once marked HIV/AIDS but presumably no longer does. For example, in a *People* magazine article commemorating what would have been Ryan's fiftieth birthday in December 2021, Joelle Goldstein wrote that "White became a symbol of hope during a time when fear and misconceptions about AIDS were prevalent in the United States."[73] But old misconceptions persist, and they've been joined by newer ones, including the notion that HIV/AIDS is somehow over (or mostly over). Just as the Ryan White story has often sharpened the lines between those who supposedly deserved HIV/AIDS and those who didn't, narratives that relegate HIV and AIDS to the past (or to Africa) obscure the fact that some populations in the United States remain particularly susceptible to infection, illness, and death. It is no accident that the burdens of HIV and AIDS, some thirty-five years after Ryan's death and the passage of the Ryan White CARE Act, continue to be borne by the most stigmatized populations in the United States—people who use intravenous drugs; queer and trans people; those without health insurance; and Black, Brown, and Indigenous people.[74]

It is also no accident that similar processes have unfolded within the COVID-19 pandemic and the mpox epidemic. While "We're All in This Together" became a rallying cry during the early phases of the coronavirus pandemic, the tolls of COVID-19 were and remain unevenly distributed.[75] Further, mpox recirculated tried-and-true tropes positioning queer people as vectors of disease. Notions of innocence and guilt, deservingness and undeservingness, and absolution and blame have defined these crises. Only by troubling and ultimately dismantling such binaries can we solve our health crises and secure a fairer, healthier, and brighter future for all people.

EPILOGUE

In response to this health crisis, the American people did as we always do: We mobilized the resources of the nation to fight this epidemic, not just in our own nation, in our communities, but ultimately in every corner of the world.

America has been on a long journey fighting this disease since it first emerged. And much of the progress that we've made here at home actually began with one young man's story—a boy from my home state of Indiana named Ryan White.

Vice President Mike Pence,
speaking at a World AIDS Day event, 2018

Beginning in late 2014 and stretching into 2015—twenty-five years after Ryan White's death and almost twenty years after Andrew Sullivan published his infamous article "When Plagues End"—the town of Austin, in Scott County, Indiana, experienced one of the largest HIV outbreaks in recent American history.[1] Some 200 people in and around Austin contracted HIV primarily by injecting the prescription opioid Opana.[2] Indiana's governor at the time, Mike Pence, faced tremendous criticism for his delayed response to the crisis and his initial unwillingness to lift the statewide ban on needle-exchange programs. Under pressure from public health leaders and elected officials from across the political spectrum, Pence eventually issued an executive order authorizing the operation of a syringe-exchange program in Scott County.[3]

The following year, Donald Trump selected Pence to serve as his running mate on the Republican presidential ticket, and in early 2020, Trump tapped Pence to lead what would be an uneven and inadequate White House response to the COVID-19 pandemic.[4] Pence's sordid public health record reveals the continuities between HIV/AIDS and COVID-19 and illustrates both the continued relevance and the limits of the Ryan White story. Indeed, even

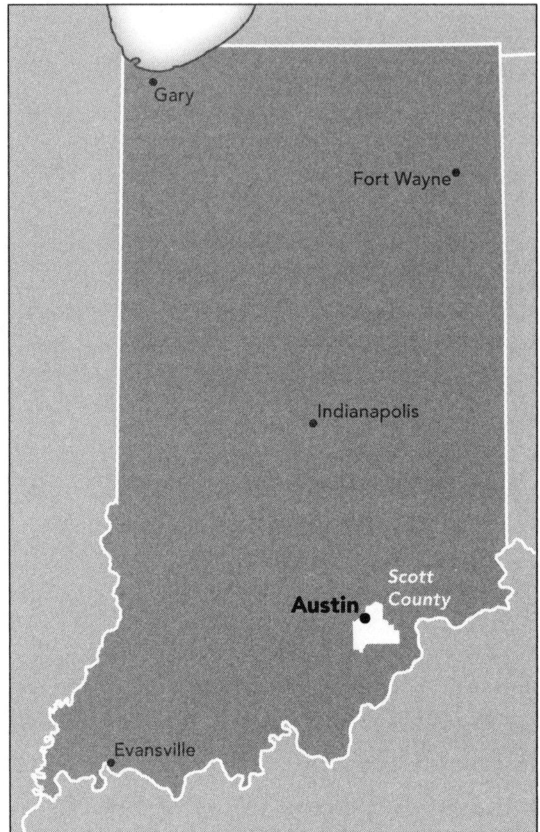

Austin, Indiana, site of the 2014–15 HIV outbreak. Map by Daniel Huffman.

as Pence has shown his hostility to certain forms of scientific knowledge, models of health care provision, and ways of being, he has also invoked the spirit of Ryan White to weave teleological narratives of medical and social progress.

PENCE'S PLAGUES

Mike Pence wanted to be in the US House of Representatives. But after running unsuccessful campaigns in 1988 and 1990 against longtime Democratic congressman Philip Sharp (who represented Indiana's Second Congressional District), Pence found his way into the world of conservative talk radio. By the mid-1990s, his daily talk show was syndicated throughout Indiana, and he hosted a weekly political television program on Indianapolis's WNDY-TV.

After boosting his profile through his radio and television presence, Pence once again ran for Congress in 2000.[5] His campaign platform, titled "The Pence Agenda: A Guide to Renewing the American Dream," sought to energize religious and social conservatives by focusing on the threats purportedly facing American families—namely queer people, people who use intravenous drugs, and people with AIDS. "The traditional two parent family is the nucleus of our civilization," Pence declared in his "Agenda." "We can renew the American dream by rekindling the fires of men, material and morale that warm the warriors who stand on liberty's ramparts protecting our families."[6]

Accordingly, as federal lawmakers worked to reauthorize the Ryan White CARE Act again in the year 2000, Pence hoped to place conditions on this proposed reauthorization and to discipline the populations deemed responsible for spreading HIV. "Congress should support the reauthorization of the Ryan White [CARE] Act only after completion of an audit to ensure that federal dollars were no longer being given to organizations that celebrate and encourage the types of behaviors that facilitate the spreading of the HIV virus," Pence's campaign platform read. "Resources should be directed toward those institutions which provide assistance to those seeking to change their sexual behavior."[7] By distinguishing between presumably innocent and guilty people with AIDS, Pence sounded many of the same notes that Jesse Helms had in his opposition to the CARE Act throughout the 1990s. Further, Pence seemed to endorse the scientifically baseless practice of conversion therapy, which promises to "cure" homosexuality.

Pence's apparent rejection of the well-documented dangers of cigarettes also became an issue during the 2000 campaign. In an editorial circulated on his campaign website, Pence wrote, "Despite the hysteria from the political class and the media, smoking doesn't kill." During a debate held in the run-up to the election, Pence's Democratic opponent, Bob Rock, confronted him about the editorial. In response, Pence explained that there was no "scientific causal link" between smoking and lung cancer. "The thrust of that article, Bob," he told his opponent, "was that we do not need a government large enough in Washington, D.C., that can protect me from myself."[8]

Pence nevertheless defeated Rock and soon thereafter began his first term as congressman. He would be reelected five times. During his twelve years in Congress, Pence demonstrated his hostility to publicly funded health care and health insurance. In 2003, for instance, he fell just short in his attempt to block President George W. Bush's Medicare expansion plan, which added a prescription drug benefit to the program.[9] Congressman

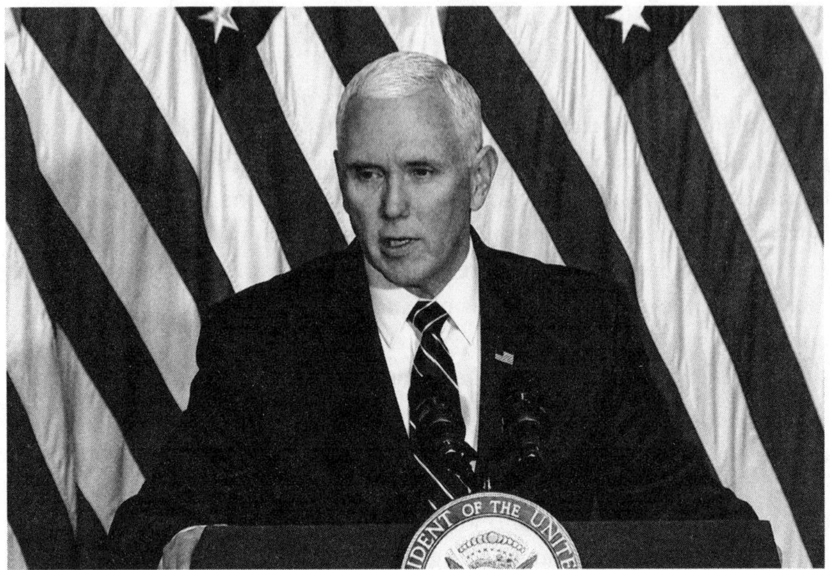

Vice President Mike Pence delivers remarks at the White House World AIDS Day Event, November 29, 2018. Trump White House Archived, YouTube, www.youtube.com/watch?v=OvmHDWieq04.

Pence also proved to be an ardent opponent of LGBTQ+ causes—resisting marriage equality, the repeal of "Don't Ask, Don't Tell," and the Employment Non-Discrimination Act.[10]

These sensibilities carried over into Pence's term as Indiana's governor from 2013 to 2017. In this role, Pence built on his predecessor Mitch Daniels's efforts to prioritize "personal responsibility" in the provision of Medicaid.[11] He also made national headlines when he signed into law the Religious Freedom Restoration Act, which ostensibly enabled the free exercise of religion but which critics claimed permitted antigay and anti-trans discrimination under the guise of "Religious Freedom." The law provoked a backlash among some business and political leaders. Apple CEO Tim Cook, who is openly gay, condemned Indiana's Religious Freedom Restoration Act, while some companies vowed to halt construction or expansion plans in the state.[12] Then came the Scott County HIV outbreak, for which Pence has never been held accountable and which did nothing to derail Pence's political career.

On the contrary, Pence soon found himself in the White House, where in 2018 he delivered a speech to mark World AIDS Day. Fellow Hoosier Ryan

White played a central role in Pence's address. For the vice president, Ryan "faced discrimination and a stigma associated with the disease, in part due to the misunderstanding about HIV/AIDS at the time." But in the end, Pence indicated, Ryan's "courage and example . . . helped educate the American people about the realities of HIV/AIDS, and it galvanized the United States Congress to act." After White's death, Pence explained, Congress "passed the Ryan White Comprehensive AIDS Resource Emergency Act [*sic*]. And his legacy lives on to this day." The audience applauded before Pence summed up Ryan's impressive legacy. "As we speak, the Ryan White CARE Act continues to provide vital medical services to more than 1.1 million people in the United States living with HIV. And since the days when Ryan White was first diagnosed, we've grown in our understanding of HIV/AIDS and our ability to turn a deadly disease into a manageable and chronic condition."[13]

Although the presumably innocent and "politically safe" Ryan White figured prominently in Pence's speech, those disproportionately affected by HIV and AIDS—queer and trans people, Black and Brown people, and those who use intravenous drugs—were nowhere to be found.[14] Pence's failure to mention these vulnerable populations reflected his long history of neglecting the dispossessed. Moreover, despite Pence's Pollyannaish and narrow understanding of HIV and AIDS history, instantiated through the figure of Ryan White, the story of HIV and AIDS remains one of inequality, suffering, and shame. "From the beginning," queer theorist Michael Warner observes, "AIDS has affected most those populations lowest in the hierarchy of respectability."[15] As a supposedly innocent person with AIDS, Ryan White occupied a much different position in the hierarchy of respectability. And although this position did not protect Ryan from infection, illness, and eventually death, he secured the sort of dignity, respect, and care that ought to be the norm for people living with HIV and AIDS. Yet it wasn't, and it still isn't.

While Pence touted "our ability to turn a deadly disease into a manageable and chronic condition" in his 2018 World AIDS Day remarks, he glossed over several damning facts.[16] First, AIDS continues to kill thousands in the United States and hundreds of thousands across the world each year. Next, HIV is hardly "manageable" for the estimated 158,500 Americans whose HIV infection remains undiagnosed, partially because of lingering stigmas.[17] And finally, profound inequalities in health care provision and health outcomes for those living with HIV and AIDS point to larger structural problems that cannot be remedied through pathbreaking research and miracle drugs alone. For instance, the rise of pre-exposure prophylaxis, or PrEP, and post-exposure prophylaxis in the 2010s offered tremendous hope for those deemed at risk of HIV infection. But the benefits of these innovations, just like the risks of HIV and AIDS, remain unevenly distributed.[18] Only 25 percent of those who indicate for PrEP are actually on it, and only 9 percent of Black people who indicate for PrEP take it.[19]

Though politically expedient, Pence's version of the Ryan White story cannot account for the fact that Black people make up just 13 percent of the US population but 41 percent of new HIV diagnoses and 52 percent of HIV-related deaths. It cannot account for the fact that Hispanic or Latinx people represent about 19 percent of the total population but 29 percent of new HIV diagnoses in the United States.[20] And it cannot account for the fact that HIV continues to affect queer and trans people at astronomical rates. Gay, bisexual, and other men who have sex with men constituted 70 percent of new HIV infections in the United States in 2019. Meanwhile, according to certain CDC estimates, some 42 percent of transgender women in the United States are HIV-positive. The numbers among Black trans women are even higher.[21]

Just fifteen months after Pence delivered his World AIDS Day remarks, and despite his deeply rooted hostility toward certain forms of medical knowledge and health care provision, he was selected to lead the White House's coronavirus task force. Suffice it to say, Pence's stint with the task force proved to be an unmitigated disaster. As hundreds of thousands of Americans died and millions more got sick, Pence did Trump's bidding, downplaying the severity of the pandemic and minimizing the need for more stringent health measures. Electoral considerations no doubt informed his decision-making on the task force. "Fighting a pandemic of this magnitude is very hard," the vice president told a staff member. "Fighting a pandemic in an election year is even harder."[22] The pandemic would eventually cost Trump and Pence the 2020 election.

But even with the ascent of a supposedly more enlightened presidential administration, one ostensibly committed to ending COVID-19, the pandemic raged on. Just like his predecessor, President Joe Biden often cast his administration's efforts to fight the pandemic in heroic terms, and at times Biden seemed to prioritize the economy over the lives of workers. While he had secured victory in the 2020 election by criticizing Trump and Pence's COVID-19 response, Biden increasingly shifted the blame toward the unvaccinated during his presidency. With the Omicron surge looming in the winter of 2021–22, he warned, "We are looking at a winter of severe illness and death for the unvaccinated."[23] Yet as effective as the COVID-19 vaccines were (and remain), they were not a panacea, and the COVID-19 death toll among vaccinated people continues to rise. Furthermore, uneven access, uptake, and eligibility—for children, undocumented people, and the immunocompromised, for instance—undermined the potential impact of the vaccines. In September 2022, President Biden prematurely declared the coronavirus pandemic "over," and in the spring of 2023, the White House dissolved its COVID-19 task force.[24]

Similar patterns emerged in the summer of 2022 and beyond as queer communities throughout the world grappled with the mpox virus, an "orthopoxvirus related to smallpox [and] endemic to Central and West Africa."[25] Epidemiologist and longtime HIV/AIDS activist Gregg Gonsalves has explained that the Biden administration "moved incredibly slowly" in response to the mpox virus, thereby missing an opportunity to "stop . . . it in its tracks."[26] As a result, activists sprang into action to demand greater federal involvement and expanded vaccine access. But when these efforts proved effective in limiting infection among certain segments of the queer community—particularly white gay men in affluent countries—some commentators prematurely declared victory. For their part, Ina Park and Dan Savage penned a *New York Times* editorial titled "How Gay Men Saved Us from Mpox" in April 2023.[27] The piece curiously implied that the mpox virus threat had dissipated—even as outbreaks continued in Africa, even as vaccines were virtually nonexistent throughout parts of the Global South, and even as communities of color bore the brunt of the epidemic in the United States.[28] According to the CDC, Black men represented 90 percent of mpox deaths in the United States between May 2022 and March 2023. The majority of those who died were immunocompromised due to HIV infection, a sobering reminder that these seemingly discrete epidemiological phenomena are actually inextricably linked.[29]

Likewise, the narratives of blame and absolution and obsolescence that have structured understandings of COVID-19 and the mpox virus mirror those used in the 1980s and 1990s HIV/AIDS epidemic. Certain iterations of Ryan White's story served to distinguish between righteous and unrighteous people with AIDS, thereby legitimating the mass death, disability, and suffering sustained at the height of the crisis. When the federal government finally addressed the epidemic in a meaningful way, it did so by harnessing the symbolic power of a beloved, uncontroversial person with AIDS at the top of various hierarchies of victimhood. Indeed, as welcome as the CARE Act was, the decision to name it after Ryan White sent a clear signal to the populations hit hardest by HIV/AIDS. Nearly three decades later, Mike Pence's decision to honor Ryan in his 2018 World AIDS Day speech—and to ignore queer and trans people, African Americans, Latinx people, and other groups—sent a similar message. And by relegating to the past the "stigma associated with the disease," Pence used Ryan White to conceal the discrimination and difficulties that so many (disproportionately Black, Brown, queer, and trans) people with HIV or AIDS still endure in the United States and beyond.

Ryan White's story should not be one of exclusion or exceptionalism. It should not serve to draw lines between the guilty and the innocent. It should not work to disparage the presumably ill-informed and celebrate the enlightened. It should not serve as a reminder of a bygone stigma—since that stigma persists, in large part because of the bigotry of people like Jesse Helms and Mike Pence.

The Ryan White story should be one of compassion. It should be a story about all people with HIV and AIDS—and the challenges they faced and continue to face. It should be a story about the sick and the healthy and the shape of care. It should be a story about the power of kinship and our responsibilities to one another. It should be a story that helps us envision another world—one in which health care is neither a privilege nor a commodity but a right, one in which sympathy and love extend not only to the "innocent," one in which the burdens of one community are the burdens of all, and one in which we carry each other. Let this be Ryan's story.

ACKNOWLEDGMENTS

This book would not have been possible without the support and encouragement of many, many people. Most of the research for this project was undertaken amid the COVID-19 pandemic, the early phases of which witnessed the temporary closure of many archives and libraries. In this moment, archivists kindly sent me relevant materials from their collections: Randy Smith and Stewart Lauterbach at the Howard County Historical Society, Richard Carney at the Jesse Helms Center Archives at Wingate University, Nathan Jones at the Vanderbilt Television News Archive, Rachael Stoeltje at the Indiana University Moving Image Archive, and archivists at the George H. W. Bush Presidential Library and Museum in Texas, the Special Collections Research Center at George Washington University, and the Division of Rare and Manuscript Collections at Cornell University.

Others provided assistance and guidance once their archives opened back up in 2021 and 2022: Carrie Lynn Schwier at the Indiana University Archives in Bloomington, Maire Gurevitz at the Indiana Historical Society, Keenan Salla at the Indiana State Archives, Stephen M. Lane at Indiana University–Purdue University Indianapolis (now two separate universities), and others. This book benefited tremendously from their hard work and generosity.

Philina Martinez, Tracy Horrell, and Della Clouse graciously allowed me to access Ron Colby's personal files in the Western Middle School Library in Russiaville. These materials proved absolutely invaluable. So too did the rich oral histories conducted by Allen Safianow, Judy Lausch, and Diane Knight under the aegis of the Howard County Historical Society. Jonathan Morgan helped me better understand the intricacies of the Ryan White HIV/AIDS Program. Lamar Wilson kindly shared his knowledge about Robert Rayford. Ted Frantz informed me of some relevant materials in the Institute for Civic Leadership and Digital Mayoral Archives at the University of Indianapolis. He also read and provided helpful feedback on an earlier draft of chapter 5.

Other friends, colleagues, and students read drafts, as well. Joe Gabriel, Will Hanley, Ted Kerr, Katherine Mooney, Stephen Pemberton, George Williamson, and the late, great Laurie Wood read and commented on various chapters. So too did members of a gender/sexuality studies writing group that met via Zoom at the height of COVID. This group included Katie Batza,

Jeff Berryhill, Salonee Bhaman, René Esparza, Gill Frank, Emily Hobson, Andrea Milne, Dan Royles, Natalie Shibley, and Lauren Sklaroff. The undergraduates in my Fall 2023 course America in the 1990s read and discussed chapters 5, 6, and 7. René Esparza kindly read the entire manuscript and offered detailed feedback. Ruth Reichard, who wrote the 2021 book *Blood and Steel: Ryan White, the AIDS Crisis, and Deindustrialization in Kokomo, Indiana*, also read the whole manuscript, as did Jason D'Amours, Allen Safianow, Trish Siplon, and the graduate students in my Fall 2023 US since 1968 course.

Audience members and my fellow panelists posed thought-provoking questions about my research at the American Political History Conference in West Lafayette, Indiana (June 2022) and the Organization of American Historians Conference in Los Angeles (April 2023). Special thanks go to Matt Lassiter, Abby Whitaker, George Aumoithe, Salonee Bhaman, Eileen Boris, James Chappel, and Beverly Gage.

The Council on Research and Creativity at Florida State University provided research support, as did the Ostrom Workshop at IU Bloomington.

This project has been enriched by the scholarship and thinking of so many individuals, including Katie Batza, Jennifer Brier, Margot Canaday, Brent Cebul, Jih-Fei Cheng, Cathy Cohen, Melinda Cooper, René Esparza, Ruthie Gilmore, Gregg Gonsalves, Colin Gordon, Linda Gordon, Deborah Gould, Evelynn Hammonds, Elizabeth Hinton, Emily Hobson, Mariame Kaba, Matt Lassiter, Erica Meiners, Bethany Moreton, Joseph Osmundson, Stephen Pemberton, Ruth Reichard, Dan Royles, Sarah Schulman, Landon Storrs, Keeanga-Yamahtta Taylor, Heather Ann Thompson, Steven Thrasher, Jackie Wang, and Lamar Wilson.

The entire team at the University of North Carolina Press has been fantastic. Brandon Proia signed this book, and even though he now works for a different press, he has supported this project every step of the way. Andreína Fernández has been an exceptional editor, providing much-needed feedback, encouragement, and guidance throughout the process. She also helped place this book in UNC Press's Gender and American Culture series, in which my graduate advisor Landon Storrs published her first book and for which Linda Kerber (Landon's predecessor at the University of Iowa) served as a cofounding series editor (with Nell Irvin Painter). The current series editors, Mary Kelley and Martha Jones, offered sharp and constructive feedback on the book manuscript. Julie Bush and Mary Carley Caviness provided superb edits. Sonya Bonczek did a wonderful job of promoting the book. Further, the three anonymous reviewers secured by UNC Press helped make this a stronger, more polished, and more nuanced book. For that, I am incredibly grateful.

Daniel Huffman created beautiful maps for this book, and Varsha Venkatasubramanian made the index. Their hard work is greatly appreciated.

I'd also like to thank my colleagues at FSU for their kindness and support. Special thanks go to Deb Alexander, Kathleen Powers Conti, Leigh Edwards, Andrew Frank, Joe Gabriel, Will Hanley, Anasa Hicks, Meegan Kennedy, Jen Koslow, Anne Kozar, Weiwei Luo, Jeanne Martin, Katherine Mooney, John Netter, James Palmer, Christine Rizzi, Madeline Robertson, Ashley Sadler, Suzy Sinke, Candace Ward, George Williamson, and Lamar Wilson. Ed Gray was a dear friend and colleague who died suddenly in December 2023. I miss him.

I'm very fortunate to play basketball twice a week with a great group that includes Trevor Bryan, Martin Coon, Lance Mitchell, the Price brothers, Esaa Mohammad Sabti Samarah, Stephen Tripodi, Cedric Tucker, the Ward brothers, and Sean Webster.

As I wrote and revised this book, I listened to a lot of Beyoncé, Day Wave, Maxo Kream, Kacey Musgraves, The National, Charlie Puth, Rostam, Troye Sivan, Sufjan Stevens, Vampire Weekend, and Waxahatchee.

My wonderful friends, family members, and neighbors encouraged and supported me during the research and writing process. In particular, I'd like to thank the Reeds, the Tripodi-Tierney family, the Bricklers, the Mullens, the Sittigs, Beth Green, Don and Sue Mills, the Freesmeiers, Lynne Quimby-Pennock, Robert Pennock, Karen Oehme, Nat Stern, the Franks, Chad Oaks, Jonathan Rigsby, Shelby Green, Durward Rackleff, John Combs, Ed Gray, Stacey Rutledge, Anasa Hicks, Eli Wilkins-Malloy, Desmond Woodrow Malloy, Michael Franklin, Dan Luedtke, David Campbell, Martin Kavka, Tip Tomberlin, Channing Frampton, Jonathan Jackson, Greg Springer, Byrd McDaniel, Clara Schwager, Ezra McDaniel, Jacob Lee, Emily Woodruff, Matt Stanley, and Ruby Woodruff-Stanley. Special thanks go to my partner, Blake; my mother and father; and my beloved dogs, Huey and Gumbo.

Above all, I want to acknowledge Ryan White, his family, and every person who has been touched by HIV and AIDS. This book is for them.

CHRONOLOGY

1971

December 6: Ryan Wayne White is born. He is diagnosed with severe hemophilia A shortly thereafter.[1]

1984

December: Ryan, at age thirteen, is diagnosed with AIDS during a prolonged hospital stay.

1985

July 30: Western School Corporation superintendent J. O. Smith bars Ryan from attending classes in person. News outlets from across the country, such as the *Los Angeles Times* and *Chicago Tribune*, begin covering Ryan's story.

August 8: White family attorney Charles Vaughan files suit in US district court, seeking to affirm Ryan's right to attend Western School Corporation schools.

August 15: About fifty Western School Corporation teachers vote in support of superintendent Smith's decision concerning Ryan White.

August 16: Federal judge James E. Noland, based in Indianapolis, indicates that the US district court cannot accept White's case until his attorneys exhaust all administrative appeals.

August 26: Classes begin at Western Middle School, though Ryan is forced to attend his classes virtually through a telephone hookup. "It stinks!" he declares in a clip broadcast on the *NBC Nightly News* and ABC's *World News Tonight* that evening.

September 19: School officials meet with Jeanne White and her attorney, Charles Vaughan, to discuss Ryan's status. Their report, released in early October, recommends that Ryan continue to learn remotely.

November 25: After hearing testimony from White's attorneys and those representing the Western School Corporation, the Indiana Department of Education rules that Ryan should be permitted to attend classes in person when he is not extremely ill.

December 17: Western's school board decides to appeal the Department of Education ruling.

1986

Early February: Ryan, Jeanne, and Andrea White visit Rome, where they appear on the television program *Italia Sera*.

February 6: The Indiana Department of Education appeals board affirms Ryan's right to attend school, so long as he is cleared by the Howard County health officer, Dr. Alan Adler. After examining Ryan the following week, Adler determines that he is healthy enough to return to school.

February 21: Ryan returns to Western Middle School amid much fanfare, but his day is spoiled by two developments. First, 42 percent of the student body stays home that day for fear of contracting HIV. Second, parents convince a Howard County judge to issue a temporary injunction preventing Ryan from attending classes in person.

March 12: Ryan's attorney files a motion requesting a change of venue for the upcoming hearing regarding the temporary injunction.

April 9: A circuit judge in the neighboring county of Clinton vacates the injunction, thereby permitting Ryan to return to Western Middle School. Later that month, over the objections of concerned Howard County parents, the same Clinton County judge upholds his earlier order.

July 18: Indiana's court of appeals rejects the concerned parents' appeal.

August 25: After the Howard County Health Department evaluates Ryan and certifies him fit to attend school, he begins the eighth grade at Western High School.

1987

Spring: After a difficult school year in which Ryan faces discrimination and multiple health scares, the White family decides to move to Cicero, a small town about thirty miles south of Kokomo. Pop star Elton John helps Jeanne purchase a home there. Ryan is also approved to take AZT (azidothymidine), an antiretroviral medication often used to treat AIDS.

August: Ryan appears on the cover of *People* magazine and starts classes at Hamilton Heights High School in Arcadia, just a few miles from his new home in Cicero.

1988

March 3: Ryan testifies before the President's Commission on the HIV Epidemic in Washington, DC.

1989

January 16: *The Ryan White Story*, a television movie based largely on Ryan's struggles in Kokomo and Russiaville, first airs on ABC. An estimated 15 million Americans tune in.

1990

Late March and early April: Ryan falls ill with what the Associated Press calls an "AIDS-related respiratory infection complicated by his hemophilia." He is admitted to Indianapolis's Riley Hospital for Children, where he remains until his death. On April 4, as Ryan clings to life, the Senate Committee on Labor and Human Resources reports favorably on S. 2240, the Comprehensive AIDS Resources Emergency Act, and decides to name the proposed bill after Ryan.

April 8: Ryan White dies at the age of eighteen. His funeral is held three days later at the Second Presbyterian Church in Indianapolis. Over 1,500 people attend, including Elton John, Michael Jackson, and First Lady Barbara Bush. The ceremony airs live on national television.

August 18: The Ryan White CARE Act, overwhelmingly approved by both houses of Congress, is signed into law by President George H. W. Bush.

1996

May 20: After a protracted struggle in Congress, President Bill Clinton formally reauthorizes the Ryan White CARE Act. The CARE Act is reauthorized again in 2000, 2006, and 2009. Although the act expired in 2013, the Ryan White HIV/AIDS Program lives on. It is the largest HIV-specific federal program, providing essential services to about half of all the people diagnosed with HIV/AIDS in the United States.

NOTES

Abbreviations Used in the Notes

ACT UP	AIDS Coalition to Unleash Power
AP	Associated Press
APP	American Presidency Project, University of California, Santa Barbara
HCHS	Howard County Historical Society, Kokomo, IN
IHS	Indiana Historical Society, Indianapolis
JHCA	Jesse Helms Center Archives, Wingate University, Wingate, NC
NGLTF	National Gay and Lesbian Task Force Records (later National LGBTQ Task Force Records [1973–2017]), Division of Rare and Manuscript Collections, Carl A. Kroch Library, Cornell University, Ithaca, NY
NGTF	National Gay Task Force Records (later National LGBTQ Task Force Records [1973–2017]), Division of Rare and Manuscript Collections, Carl A. Kroch Library, Cornell University, Ithaca, NY
RWOHP	Ryan White Oral History Project, Howard County Historical Society, Kokomo, IN
UPI	United Press International
VTNA	Vanderbilt Television News Archive, Vanderbilt University, Nashville, TN
WMS	Personal Files of Ron Colby, Western Middle School Library Collection, Russiaville, IN
WSJV	WSJV News Collection (ABC 28, Elkhart/South Bend, IN), Moving Image Archive, Indiana University Libraries, Bloomington

Introduction

1. Gran Fury, *All People with AIDS Are Innocent* (1988), Whitney Museum of American Art, New York City, gift of Gran Fury.
2. Lowery, *It Was Vulgar and It Was Beautiful*, 5.
3. Dudley Clendinen, "'Epidemic of Fear' in US Schools," *New York Times*, September 8, 1985, 1; *NBC Nightly News*, August 16, 1985, record no. 545304, VTNA. See also Brier, "'Save Our Kids, Keep AIDS Out.'"
4. *NBC Nightly News*, August 26, 1985, record no. 545514, VTNA; "AIDS Quarantine," *Indianapolis Star*, January 5, 1987, 6; Raymond Guterman, "Ryan White Became a Friend in Spirit to Many," *Tampa Bay Times*, May 23, 1990. For "poster child," see (among many other examples) Ashcraft, interview, RWOHP.
5. For contemporaneous analysis of Ryan White's "innocence," see "'Innocent Victim' Ryan White Dies," *New Works News* (Indianapolis) 9, no. 8 (May 1990): 5; series 1: Periodicals, HQ 75.W62, M 1242, Michael Bohr Collection, Indy Pride Chris Gonzalez Library and Archives (ca. 1960s–2016), Manuscript and Visual Collections Department, William Henry Smith Memorial Library, IHS.
6. Patton, *Fatal Advice*.
7. Ronald Reagan, "'We Owe It to Ryan,'" *Washington Post*, April 11, 1990, A23, www.washingtonpost.com/archive/opinions/1990/04/11/we-owe-it-to-ryan/5d132882-b7e5-48dc-950c-e91003f1a690/.
8. For more on the narrow understanding of "AIDS education" that developed in the 1980s, see Patton, *Fatal Advice*.
9. Reagan, "'We Owe It to Ryan.'"
10. Gould, *Moving Politics*, esp. chap. 2. For more on "organized abandonment," see the work of geographers David Harvey and Ruth Wilson Gilmore.
11. Cohen, *Boundaries of Blackness*.
12. Petro, *After the Wrath of God*, 2.
13. Susan F. Rasky, "How the Politics Shifted on AIDS Funds," *New York Times*, May 20, 1990, 22.
14. Warner, *Trouble with Normal*, 197.
15. Cheng, Juhasz, and Shahani, "Preface," xviii.
16. "Dispatches on the Globalizations of AIDS," 52.
17. Quoted in Brent Larkin, "Kokomo Can Breathe Now, Ryan's Dead," *Cleveland Plain Dealer*, n.d. [April 1990], WMS.
18. Royles, *To Make the Wounded Whole*; Steven W. Thrasher, "The US Has an HIV Epidemic—And Its Victims Are Gay Black Men," *The Guardian*, May 30, 2018, www.theguardian.com/commentisfree/2018/may/30/black-gay-men-aids-hiv-epidemic-america.
19. The literature on whiteness is too voluminous to cite in its entirety, but key works include Roediger, *Wages of Whiteness*; Ignatiev, *How the Irish Became White*; Du Bois, *Black Reconstruction in America*; Lipsitz, *Possessive Investment in Whiteness*; Jacobson, *Whiteness of a Different Color*; HoSang, *Racial Propositions*; and Painter, *History of White People*. For critiques of whiteness studies

and the history of whiteness, see Arnesen, "Whiteness and the Historians' Imagination"; Fields, "Whiteness, Racism, and Identity"; and Kolchin, "Whiteness Studies."

20. Cheng, Juhasz, and Shahani, "Preface," xxiv.
21. Mackenzie, *Structural Intimacies*, 48 (emphasis added).
22. "AIDS: We Are Not Immune," *Emerge* 2, no. 2 (November 1990): 30–44. "Children," in this instance, were defined as those under the age of thirteen.
23. Quoted in Cheng, Juhasz, and Shahani, "Introduction," 11.
24. Hobson and Royles, "AIDS Crisis Is Not Over." Histories of HIV/AIDS published in this period include Carroll, *Mobilizing New York*; Petro, *After the Wrath of God*; Stewart-Winter, *Queer Clout*; Hobson, *Lavender and Red*; Mumford, *Not Straight, Not White*; McKay, *Patient Zero and the Making of the AIDS Epidemic*; Bost, *Evidence of Being*; Bell, *Beyond the Politics of the Closet*; Royles, *To Make the Wounded Whole*; Chávez, *Borders of AIDS*; Vider, *Queerness of Home*; and Canaday, *Queer Career*.
25. "Interchange."
26. In the only other monograph focused on the subject, Ruth Reichard considers the Ryan White story alongside Kokomo's experience with deindustrialization. Reichard, *Blood and Steel*.
27. Patton, "Foreword," ix.
28. Resnik, *Blood Saga*, 32.
29. See Thrasher, *Viral Underclass*.
30. "Track Covid-19 in the US," *New York Times*, updated March 26, 2024, www.nytimes.com/interactive/2023/us/covid-cases.html.
31. See especially Ina Park and Dan Savage, "How Gay Men Saved Us from Mpox," *New York Times*, April 16, 2023, www.nytimes.com/2023/04/16/opinion/gay-men-mpox.html.

Chapter One

1. White with Dworkin, *Weeding Out the Tears*, 37, 38, 40.
2. White and Cunningham, *Ryan White*, 3.
3. For examples of this formulation ("through no fault of his own") in Ryan's case, see the following in the RWOHP: Carter, interview; Ferries, interview; Lawson, interview; and Rosselot, interview.
4. White with Dworkin, *Weeding Out the Tears*, 49, 74.
5. Sturken, *Tangled Memories*, 150.
6. Minutes, "Meeting of the Ad Hoc A.I.D. Task Force," July 14, 1982, box 118, folder 14 (Hemophiliacs, 1982–85), NGTF. The organization changed its name to the National Gay and Lesbian Task Force (NGLTF) in 1985. This name appears later in the book.
7. For examples of the "AIDS victim" formulation, see "AIDS Boy Loses Round," *Los Angeles Times*, August 16, 1985, 1; "AIDS Victim Called to Classes," *Chicago Tribune*, August 27, 1985, 8; Amory Paine, "Ryan White Wins Court Battle,"

The Advocate (Indiana Civil Liberties Union) 3, no. 1 (Spring 1986): 1, object no. 2013.0181.004, box 1, folder 3, OMB 0138, Series 1: Newsletters, ACLU of Indiana Records (1953–2013), Manuscript and Visual Collections Department, William Henry Smith Memorial Library, IHS; *NBC Nightly News*, August 31, 1987, record no. 558073, VTNA.

8. Resnik, *Blood Saga*, 8, 12, 18; Pemberton, *Bleeding Disease*, 21, 79.
9. Resnik, *Blood Saga*, 40, 47.
10. Joe Frolik, "Hemophiliac's Lifeline May Also Be a Danger," *Cleveland Plain Dealer*, March 14, 1983, 1B, box 118, folder 14, NGTF.
11. Resnik, *Blood Saga*, chap. 5.
12. Resnik, *Blood Saga*, 70; "'Special-Education' Status Eyed for Ryan," *Indianapolis Star*, September 19, 1985, 23. See also "AIDS Lawyer Plans Change in Tactics," *Kokomo (IN) Tribune*, August 19, 1985, 1; "AIDS Victim in Good Condition," *Chicago Tribune*, September 30, 1985, 3.
13. Jack Friedman and Bill Shaw, "Amazing Grace," *People*, May 30, 1988.
14. Cheng, "Cold Blood," 143, 144; Resnik, *Blood Saga*, 32. See also Pépin, *Origins of AIDS*. My thanks go to one of the external reviewers for the recommendation.
15. Davidson, *Concerto for the Left Hand*, 35.
16. Frolik, "Hemophiliac's Lifeline May Also Be a Danger."
17. Gilbert C. White and Henry R. Lesesne, "Hemophilia, Hepatitis, and the Acquired Immunodeficiency Syndrome," *Annals of Internal Medicine* 98, no. 3 (March 1, 1983): 403–4; Institute of Medicine, *HIV and the Blood Supply*, 158, quoted in Siplon, *AIDS and the Policy Struggle in the United States*, 51.
18. White with Dworkin, *Weeding Out the Tears*, 61.
19. Frolik, "Hemophiliac's Lifeline May Also Be a Danger."
20. Jerry Schwartz, "AIDS Scare Convulses Lifestyles," AP, n.d. [likely June 1983], n.p., box 118, folder 14, NGTF. For another version of this article, see Jerry Schwartz, "Targets of AIDS Disease Forced to Make Hard Choices," *Orange Coast (CA) Daily Pilot*, June 30, 1983, A8.
21. Schwartz, "AIDS Scare Convulses Lifestyles"; Frolik, "Hemophiliac's Lifeline May Also Be a Danger."
22. The title of this section comes from Stephen Kulieke, "NGTF, Others Decry Gay Blood Ban by National Hemophilia Group," *The Advocate*, March 3, 1983, box 118, folder 14, NGTF. "I don't have to tell you what 'gay blood, bad blood' could mean to a community that has historically been discriminated against, particularly in employment," NGTF executive director Virginia Apuzzo told *The Advocate*. Lawrence K. Altman, "Rare Cancer Seen in 41 Homosexuals," *New York Times*, July 3, 1981, A20; minutes, "Meeting of the Ad Hoc A.I.D. Task Force with James Curran," July 13, 1982, Annenberg Memorial Building, Mount Sinai Hospital, New York City, box 118, folder 14, NGTF.
23. Minutes, "Meeting of the Ad Hoc A.I.D. Task Force with James Curran," July 13, 1982, NGTF.
24. Minutes, "Meeting of the Ad Hoc A.I.D. Task Force," July 14, 1982, NGTF.
25. See, for one, Farmer, *AIDS and Accusation*.

26. Faria et al., "Early Spread and Epidemic Ignition of HIV-1 in Human Populations."
27. Epstein, *Impure Science*, 50, 48.
28. Lawrence K. Altman, "New Homosexual Disorder Worries Health Officials," *New York Times*, May 11, 1982, C1; Epstein, *Impure Science*, 55.
29. Hobson and Royles, "Editors' Introduction," 4; Cheng, "Cold Blood."
30. McKay, *Patient Zero and the Making of the AIDS Epidemic*; McKay, "'Patient Zero'"; Tomso, "HIV Monsters." Randy Shilts's 1987 tome *And the Band Played On* helped popularize the ahistorical "Patient Zero" narrative.
31. Michael Warner, "Unsafe: Why Gay Men Are Having Risky Sex," *Village Voice*, January 31, 1995, 35, quoted in Sturken, *Tangled Memories*, 165.
32. "Opportunistic Infections and Kaposi's Sarcoma among Haitians in the United States," *Morbidity and Mortality Weekly Report* 31, no. 26 (July 9, 1982), www.cdc.gov/mmwr/preview/mmwrhtml/00001123.htm.
33. "Epidemiologic Notes and Reports: Pneumocystis carinii Pneumonia among Persons with Hemophilia A," *Morbidity and Mortality Weekly Report* 31, no. 27 (July 16, 1982), www.cdc.gov/mmwr/preview/mmwrhtml/00001126.htm.
34. Epstein, *Impure Science*, 56.
35. Philip J. Hilts, "Strange Disease Now Spreading to Hemophiliacs," *Washington Post*, July 16, 1982, box 118, folder 14, NGTF; C. A. Caceres, letter to the editor, *Washington Post*, July 24, 1982, box 118, folder 14, NGTF (emphasis in original).
36. Bryant, *Anita Bryant Story*, 62, quoted in Frank, "'Civil Rights of Parents,'" 127.
37. See Bayer, "Gays and the Stigma of Bad Blood."
38. Minutes, "Meeting of the Ad Hoc A.I.D. Task Force with James Curran," July 13, 1982, NGTF.
39. Minutes, "Meeting of the Ad Hoc A.I.D. Task Force with James Curran," July 13, 1982, NGTF; minutes, "Meeting of the Ad Hoc A.I.D. Task Force," July 14, 1982, NGTF; Andriote, *Victory Deferred*, 56.
40. Minutes, "Meeting of the Ad Hoc A.I.D. Task Force with James Curran," July 13, 1982, NGTF; minutes, "Meeting of the Ad Hoc A.I.D. Task Force," July 14, 1982, NGTF; Hilts, "Strange Disease Now Spreading to Hemophiliacs."
41. National Hemophilia Foundation Medical and Scientific Advisory Council, "Recommendations to Prevent AIDS in Patients with Hemophilia," January 14, 1983, box 111, folder 49 (Blood—Hemophilia, 1985), NGTF; National Hemophilia Foundation, "Hemophilia Newsnotes—Acquired Immune Deficiency Syndrome: National Hemophilia Foundation Doctors Issue Position," press release, January 17, 1983, box 111, folder 49, NGTF; Bayer, "Science, Politics, and the End of the Lifelong Gay Blood Donor Ban."
42. Paul Jacobs, "US Seeks to Halt Spread of New Disease," *Los Angeles Times*, March 4, 1983, B3.
43. Kulieke, "NGTF, Others Decry Gay Blood Ban by National Hemophilia Group."
44. Roger W. Enlow and Bruce R. Voeller to NGTF, "Current State of A.I.D.S. & Blood Products," January 10, 1983, box 118, folder 14, NGTF.
45. Karlis Streips, "Hemophilia Group Calls for Gay Blood Ban," *GayLife* (Chicago), January 27, 1983, box 118, folder 14, NGTF.

46. Bayer, "Science, Politics, and the End of the Lifelong Gay Blood Donor Ban."
47. Siplon, *AIDS and the Policy Struggle in the United States*, 58, 52, 53.
48. Reichard, *Blood and Steel*, 41–42.
49. Institute of Medicine, *HIV and the Blood Supply*, 194, quoted in Siplon, *AIDS and the Policy Struggle in the United States*, 58.
50. As late as November 1983, for example, the National Hemophilia Foundation released an advisory statement that read, in part, "It is important to note that only a fraction of one percent of all hemophiliacs have contracted AIDS and no common lots have been identified among those who have the disease. This strongly suggests that the great majority of people with hemophilia are not susceptible to AIDS." National Hemophilia Foundation, "Hemophilia Information Exchange—AIDS Update: Advisory no. 11," November 2, 1983, box 118, folder 14, NGTF. See also Resnik, *Blood Saga*, esp. chap. 9.
51. Resnik, *Blood Saga*, 131, 132; Frolik, "Hemophiliac's Lifeline May Also Be a Danger"; National Hemophilia Foundation, "Hemophilia Newsnotes—Medical Bulletin #4, Chapter Advisory #5, AIDS: Implications Regarding Blood Product Use; and Summary of National Hemophilia Foundation Activities," December 21, 1982, box 111, folder 49, NGTF; Jeremy Pearce, "Oscar Ratnoff, 91, Expert on Blood Clots, Is Dead," *New York Times*, June 6, 2008, www.nytimes.com/2008/06/06/health/06ratnoff.html.
52. National Hemophilia Foundation, "Hemophilia Information Exchange—AIDS Update: Advisory no. 11."
53. Reichard, *Blood and Steel*, 42.
54. Mike Schumann, "Indiana's Series with Kansas Has Seen National Titles, Heartbreak, and Instant Classics," *Daily Hoosier*, December 16, 2022, www.thedailyhoosier.com/indianas-series-with-kansas-has-seen-national-titles-heartbreak-and-instant-classics/.
55. White with Dworkin, *Weeding Out the Tears*, 40.
56. Brett, "Experience of Disability from the Perspective of Parents of Children with Profound Impairment," 828.
57. White and Cunningham, *Ryan White*, 19, 22 (emphasis in original).
58. White with Dworkin, *Weeding Out the Tears*, 42.
59. Passanante Elman, *Chronic Youth*, 23.
60. *I Have AIDS: A Teenager's Story.*
61. Petro, *After the Wrath of God*, 2.
62. White and Cunningham, *Ryan White*, 22.
63. White with Dworkin, *Weeding Out the Tears*, 48, 41.
64. White and Cunningham, *Ryan White*, 22, 22–23, 23; White with Dworkin, *Weeding Out the Tears*, 46, 48, 43.
65. White with Dworkin, *Weeding Out the Tears*, 46–47.
66. White and Cunningham, *Ryan White*, 47–48.
67. Beverly Beyette, "Life Without Ryan: Her Son Is Dead, the Media Are Gone and Jeanne White Is Putting Her Life Back Together," *Los Angeles Times*, July 15, 1990, www.latimes.com/archives/la-xpm-1990-07-15-vw-550-story.html.

68. White and Cunningham, *Ryan White*, 41, 49; White with Dworkin, *Weeding Out the Tears*, 61, 63–64.
69. Shimona Starling, "The Levee Breaks—Initial Reports of AIDS," *Nature*, November 29, 2018, www.nature.com/articles/d42859-018-00002-y.
70. White and Cunningham, *Ryan White*, 53, 57; White with Dworkin, *Weeding Out the Tears*, 73.
71. White and Cunningham, *Ryan White*, 69.
72. Press release, Detective Sergeant Roger Smith, Howard County Sheriff's Department, Criminal Investigations Division, January 20, 1989, object no. 2011.012.007–1a, HCHS; Bagby, interview, RWOHP; Bilodeau, interview, RWOHP; Ferries, interview, RWOHP; Genovese, interview, RWOHP; Johnson, interview, RWOHP. See also Steve Marschand, "Local Youth Faces AIDS," *Kokomo Tribune*, March 3, 1985, 3. Jeanne White's book does briefly state that her "friends at Delco had taken up a collection" for the White family following the Christmastime robbery. White with Dworkin, *Weeding Out the Tears*, 78.
73. White and Cunningham, *Ryan White*, 69, 47 (emphasis in original).
74. White and Cunningham, *Ryan White*, 70, 71; White with Dworkin, *Weeding Out the Tears*, 74.
75. For more on hemophilia and "normality," see Pemberton, *Bleeding Disease*; Pemberton, "Curious Case of the 'Professional Hemophiliac.'"
76. Marschand, "Local Youth Faces AIDS."
77. Ron Colby to Russell Able, August 9, 1985, WMS.
78. Paul N. Eilers, letter to the editor, *Indianapolis Star*, December 6, 1985, 25.
79. White and Cunningham, *Ryan White*, 71.
80. Rex Redifer, "Death Claims a Quiet Hero," *Indianapolis Star*, April 14, 1990, A12; Price, *The Quiet Hero*.

Chapter Two

1. For "normal kid," see Price, *Quiet Hero*, 52; and Olivier to Ryan White, March 24, 1986, Ryan White Letters, Digital Collections, Indiana University Indianapolis Library, https://iuidigital.contentdm.oclc.org/digital/collection/RyanWhite/id/23669/rec/1.
2. Steve Marschand, "Local Youth Faces AIDS," *Kokomo Tribune*, March 3, 1985, 3.
3. Christopher M. MacNeil, "School Bars Door to Youth with AIDS," *Kokomo Tribune*, July 31, 1985, 1.
4. *NBC Nightly News*, August 26, 1985, record no. 545514, VTNA; "AIDS Victim, 13, Fights Ban by School," *Chicago Tribune*, August 6, 1985, 4; ABC, *Nightline*, July 31, 1985, record no. 657094, VTNA. As Ruth Reichard writes, "Kokomo residents fell into three camps" in the Ryan White saga: "a passionately outspoken minority who feared that one undersized teenager could contaminate an entire school by his mere presence; a much quieter minority who believed strongly that the youth should be allowed to attend classes; and a very silent majority whose

beliefs, prejudices, fears, and inclinations went virtually unrecorded." Reichard, *Blood and Steel*, 2.

5. For "regular kid," see Colby, interview, RWOHP. "He didn't want special attention," Colby recalled, and "he didn't want to be singled out." Ryan "just wanted to be what everybody else was."
6. AP, "School Is Among 'Angels' Honored for AIDS Work," *Indianapolis Star*, December 9, 1995, n.p., folder 8: Clippings, Ryan White (ca. 1990s), box 8, M 1242, Michael Bohr Collection, Indy Pride Chris Gonzalez Library and Archives (ca. 1960s–2016), Manuscript and Visual Collections Department, William Henry Smith Memorial Library, IHS.
7. During one meeting of "concerned parents," the *Kokomo Tribune* noted, several parents even insisted that their "knowledge about AIDS would surpass some experts' knowledge." Christopher M. MacNeil, "Avoid Boycott, Parents Are Told," *Kokomo Tribune*, December 5, 1985, 3.
8. Elementary School Attendance and Scholarship Record, Ryan W. White, Tri-Central Community Schools (Sharpsville, IN), WMS; Ryan White, Grade 7 Scholastic Report, 1984–85 (first semester), WMS.
9. Educational Evaluation Referral, Kokomo Area Special Education Cooperative, August 23, 1985, WMS.
10. Ron Colby, questionnaire responses, n.d., WMS.
11. Carter, interview, RWOHP.
12. MacNeil, "School Bars Door to Youth with AIDS," 1.
13. "Guidelines for Children with AIDS/ARC Attending School," Indiana State Board of Health, July 30, 1985, WMS.
14. MacNeil, "School Bars Door to Youth with AIDS"; "Outrage Should Be Tempered," *Durham (NC) Morning Herald*, August 9, 1985, n.p., object no. 2012.073.0005-12, Ryan White Collection, HCHS.
15. Christopher M. MacNeil and Ann Nolan, "Guide Leaves Voids," *Kokomo Tribune*, August 1, 1985, 1.
16. *CBS Evening News*, July 31, 1985, record no. 305039, VTNA.
17. Christopher M. MacNeil, "Western Board Backs AIDS Stand," *Kokomo Tribune*, August 1, 1985, 1.
18. "Guidelines for Children with AIDS/ARC Attending School"; Western School Corporation, questions submitted to ISBH and Ryan's doctor, August 5, 1985, WMS.
19. MacNeil, "Western Board Backs AIDS Stand"; "Every Right," *Kokomo Tribune*, August 2, 1985, 5; "AIDS Case a Drain to School Finances," *Kokomo Tribune*, December 18, 1985, 1.
20. Denise Kalette, Mark Spearman, and Steven Findlay, "New Testing Would Save Other Kids," *USA Today*, August 1, 1985, 1A. For more about these precautions—and larger concerns about implementing them in Western School Corporation schools—see Colby, interview, RWOHP.
21. Carol Elrod, "AIDS: Now a Household Word, It's Invading 'Straight' World," *Indianapolis Star*, August 4, 1985, 1A. See also Mark Nichols, "Interested ICLU Sees

Ryan's Case as One of Discrimination," *Indianapolis Star*, August 4, 1985, 22A. Around the same time, former Georgia governor Lester Maddox announced that he may have acquired HIV "from contaminated blood-derived drugs" used to fight cancer. He eventually learned that he did not, in fact, have HIV. See UPI, "Lester Maddox Fears AIDS," *Los Angeles Times*, July 30, 1985, 3.

22. UPI, "Hudson Has AIDS, His Spokesman Says," *Chicago Tribune*, July 26, 1985, 5.
23. Elrod, "AIDS: Now a Household Word, It's Invading 'Straight' World."
24. Carter, interview, RWOHP.
25. "Case in the Spotlight," *Kokomo Tribune*, August 1, 1985, 1.
26. Susan O'Brien to J. O. Smith, August 30, 1985, object nos. 2012.073.0003–15a and 2012.073.0003–15b, HCHS.
27. Jane Tan to Ryan White, September 24, 1985, Ryan White Letters, Digital Collections, Indiana University Indianapolis, https://iuidigital.contentdm.oclc.org/digital/collection/RyanWhite/id/23720/rec/1.
28. Irene M. Holleran to J. O. Smith, August 5, 1985, object no. 2012.073.0003–9a, HCHS.
29. For more on the "national pedagogy" related to AIDS, see Patton, *Fatal Advice*.
30. Ina J. Sherman to J. O. Smith, August 27, 1985, object no. 2012.073.0003–14a–14e, HCHS (emphasis in original). See also Cristine Russell, "AIDS Virus Found in Patient's Tears," *Washington Post*, August 16, 1985, www.washingtonpost.com/archive/politics/1985/08/16/aids-virus-found-in-patients-tears/828fd49f-81d7–4f56–9256-d8ffbe5decca/; and Bart Barnes, "Obituaries," *Washington Post*, August 12, 1986, www.washingtonpost.com/archive/local/1986/08/12/obituaries/cd83cc13–3c2f-45e4-a455-b407ad6de4e3/.
31. O'Brien to Smith, August 30, 1985, HCHS.
32. Christopher M. MacNeil, "Some Support Gels for Western Schools," *Kokomo Tribune*, August 7, 1985, 1.
33. Kay Bacon, "Worried Parents Attend Meeting," *Kokomo Tribune*, August 13, 1985, 1. See also Christopher M. MacNeil, "Teachers Support Smith's Decision," *Kokomo Tribune*, August 16, 1985, n.p.
34. Bacon, "Worried Parents Attend Meeting." It is unclear whether Johnson was addressing the crowd gathered in the high school cafeteria or whether she was speaking directly to a *Tribune* reporter covering the meeting.
35. Ronald Reagan, remarks at a White House press briefing, September 17, 1985, Ronald Reagan Presidential Library and Museum, Simi Valley, California, reaganlibrary.gov/research/speeches/91785c. For video of the press conference, see "President Reagan's Press Conference in the East Room on September 17, 1985," Reagan Library, uploaded to YouTube on January 23, 2017, www.youtube.com/watch?v=HUk4JU85nFw.
36. Marlene Cimons, "Health Experts Glad Reagan Cited AIDS," *Los Angeles Times*, September 19, 1985, 18.
37. For Jeanne White's aversion to suing Western School Corporation, see MacNeil, "School Bars Door to Youth with AIDS." "Legal action? I don't know," Jeanne said. "We've been through so much already . . . that I think I'll let it set awhile."

38. Christopher M. MacNeil, "AIDS Suit Filed," *Kokomo Tribune*, August 8, 1985, 1.
39. "Ryan's Lawsuit Stalls," *Kokomo Tribune*, August 16, 1985, 1.
40. AP, "Conference Set in Ryan's Case," *Kokomo Tribune*, September 17, 1985, n.p.
41. Reichard, *Blood and Steel*, 73.
42. *NBC Nightly News*, August 16, 1985, record no. 545304, VTNA.
43. Reichard, *Blood and Steel*, 73.
44. Handwritten notes, case conference, September 19, 1985, WMS.
45. Ron Colby to J. O. Smith, case conference opinion, September 26, 1985, WMS.
46. Christopher M. MacNeil, "Recommendation Not Surprising," *Kokomo Tribune*, October 2, 1985, 2; Christopher M. MacNeil, "Ryan's Attorney Ready for Next Step," *Kokomo Tribune*, October 5, 1985, 1.
47. MacNeil, "Ryan's Attorney Ready for Next Step."
48. Colby to Smith, case conference opinion, WMS (emphasis in original).
49. Christopher M. MacNeil, "Western Patrons Solidify Support," *Kokomo Tribune*, September 26, 1985, 4.
50. "White's Condition Slowly Improving," *Kokomo Tribune*, October 15, 1985, 3.
51. Handwritten notes, case conference, WMS.
52. UPI, "AIDS Victim Starts School over Telephone," *New York Times*, August 27, 1985, A19.
53. *NBC Nightly News*, August 26, 1985, record no. 545514, VTNA; ABC, *World News Tonight*, August 26, 1985, record no. 98027, VTNA.
54. ABC, *World News Tonight*, August 26, 1985, VTNA.
55. "Homebound Boy Spurs Teleconferencing Aid," *Telcoms: Teleconferencing Newsletter* 8, no. 9 (September 1985): 1, WMS.
56. Handwritten notes, case conference, WMS.
57. Colby to Smith, case conference opinion, WMS.
58. "Back to 'School,'" *Kokomo Tribune*, November 14, 1985, 1. After Smith's initial decision barring Ryan from WMS, the *Kokomo Tribune*'s editorial board declared that Ryan had "every right to attend." See "Every Right."
59. "White's Lawyer Files Appeal," *Kokomo Tribune*, October 10, 1985, 3; "White's Appeal Set for Nov. 1," *Kokomo Tribune*, October 14, 1985, 3.
60. Christopher M. MacNeil, "Tempers Flare at AIDS Hearing," *Kokomo Tribune*, November 2, 1985, 1.
61. David R. Day to J. O. Smith, November 7, 1985, WMS. For analysis of this term ("best interests"), especially as it relates to children, see Briggs, *Somebody's Children*.
62. David R. Day to J. O. Smith, November 22, 1985 (post-hearing brief enclosed), WMS.
63. David R. Day to J. O. Smith and Stephen M. Jessup re: "Ryan White," November 25, 1985 (hearing examiner's decision enclosed), WMS.
64. UPI, "'Great' Present for AIDS Boy," *New York Times*, November 27, 1985, B7, www.nytimes.com/1985/11/27/us/great-present-for-aids-boy.html.
65. Barb Albert, "'Yea! I'm Going Back to School,' AIDS Kid Shouts after Ruling," *Indianapolis Star*, November 26, 1985, 1.

66. *NBC Nightly News*, November 26, 1985, record no. 540940, VTNA.
67. Christopher M. MacNeil, "Will Western Appeal Decision?," *Kokomo Tribune*, December 1, 1985, 8; "AIDS Case a Drain to School Finances."
68. "Western Appeal to Be Later," *Kokomo Tribune*, December 3, 1985, 3.
69. Dawne Slater, "Western Agenda Is Media Event," *Kokomo Tribune*, December 18, 1985, 1.
70. Christopher M. MacNeil, "14th Birthday Closes Out 'Hectic' Year for Ryan," *Kokomo Tribune*, December 7, 1985, 3.
71. Christopher M. MacNeil, "Christmas Comes Early for Ryan," *Kokomo Tribune*, December 20, 1985, 2.
72. Jennings Parrott, "Italian TV Getting an Expert to Discuss AIDS Problem," *Los Angeles Times*, January 3, 1986, 2.
73. "AIDS Victim Now a Celebrity," *Chicago Tribune*, January 4, 1986, 3.
74. UPI, "Italy Opens Heart to Indiana Boy with AIDS," *Chicago Tribune*, February 5, 1986, 3.
75. *NBC Nightly News*, February 5, 1986, record no. 548652, VTNA; AP, "Romans Lend Ryan an Ear," *Kokomo Tribune*, February 4, 1986, 1.
76. *CBS Evening News*, February 5, 1986, record no. 308572, VTNA; UPI, "Italy Opens Heart to Indiana Boy with AIDS."

Chapter Three

1. Christopher M. MacNeil, "Whites Keeping the Media Busy," *Kokomo Tribune*, February 6, 1986, 3.
2. "Epidemiologic Notes and Reports: *Pneumocystis* Pneumonia—Los Angeles," *Morbidity and Mortality Weekly Report* 30, no. 21 (June 5, 1981): 1–3.
3. "AIDS: We Are Not Immune," *Emerge* 2, no. 2 (November 1990): 30–44.
4. For more on the "national pedagogy," see Patton, *Fatal Advice*. For "hierarchy of victimhood," see Petro, *After the Wrath of God*, 2.
5. See, for example, Philip J. Hilts, "Strange Disease Now Spreading to Hemophiliacs," *Washington Post*, July 16, 1982, box 118, folder 14, NGTF.
6. See especially Sturken, *Tangled Memories*, 151–52.
7. "Drive Starts," *Kokomo Tribune*, March 17, 1973, 2.
8. Cheng, "Cold Blood"; Kerr, "How to Live with a Virus," 111.
9. Juhasz and Kerr, *We Are Having This Conversation Now*, xiii.
10. Faria et al., "Early Spread and Epidemic Ignition of HIV-1 in Human Populations."
11. Grmek, *History of AIDS*, 121.
12. Gina Kolata, "Boy's 1969 Death Suggests AIDS Invaded US Several Times," *New York Times*, October 28, 1987, A15.
13. John Crewdson, "Case Shakes Theories of AIDS Origin," *Chicago Tribune*, October 25, 1987.
14. Kolata, "Boy's 1969 Death Suggests AIDS Invaded US Several Times"; Crewdson, "Case Shakes Theories of AIDS Origin."

15. For more on St. Louis's place at the center of these historical processes, see W. Johnson, *Broken Heart of America.*
16. Cheng, "Cold Blood," 144.
17. Ayala and Spieldenner, "HIV Is a Story First Written on the Bodies of Gay and Bisexual Men."
18. Hammonds, "Race, Sex, AIDS," 28. For "white man's disease," see Royles, *To Make the Wounded Whole*, 21.
19. Crewdson, "Case Shakes Theories of AIDS Origin." For more on the disproportionate impact of HIV/AIDS on communities of color, see Cohen, *Boundaries of Blackness*; and Royles, *To Make the Wounded Whole.*
20. Many thanks to Ted Kerr for reading and commenting on this section and for his wonderful, much-needed research on Rayford's life and legacy. Thank you to L. Lamar Wilson for his work in this space as well.
21. Des Jarlais and Semaan, "HIV Prevention for Injecting Drug Users."
22. Phillips-Fein, *Fear City*; Kohler-Hausmann, *Getting Tough*; Murch, "Who's to Blame for Mass Incarceration?"
23. Des Jarlais et al., "HIV Infection among Persons Who Inject Drugs."
24. Paone et al., "New York City Syringe Exchange"; Des Jarlais et al., "HIV Infection among Persons Who Inject Drugs."
25. Kerr, "How to Live with a Virus," 111.
26. Peter Freiberg, "Thousands March Nationwide to Demand Federal Action on AIDS," *The Advocate*, June 9, 1983, 8; Allen White, "Candles and Tears on Castro: 1,000 Mourn Bobbi Campbell," *Bay Area Reporter*, August 23, 1984.
27. *CBS Evening News*, May 18, 1983, record no. 290354, VTNA; PBS, *Inside Story: Good Copy . . . Bad Medicine?*, February 17, 1984, record no. 907314, VTNA; "Gay America: Sex, Politics and the Impact of AIDS," *Newsweek*, August 8, 1983; White, "Candles and Tears on Castro."
28. Bobbi Campbell, diary entry, August 8, 1983, Bobbi Campbell Diary, MS 96–33, Special Collections, University of California, San Francisco Libraries, Online Archive of California.
29. "Gay America."
30. Wright, "Only Your Calamity."
31. Petro, *After the Wrath of God*, 2.
32. Adler, interview, RWOHP.
33. Christopher M. MacNeil, "White Decision Comes Thursday," *Kokomo Tribune*, February 11, 1986, 2; Christopher M. MacNeil, "Ryan's Schooling Is Medically OK," *Kokomo Tribune*, February 14, 1986.
34. MacNeil, "Ryan's Schooling Is Medically OK"; Christopher M. MacNeil, "Western Plans No Further Action," *Kokomo Tribune*, February 14, 1986, 10. See also Alan J. Adler, written permit, February 13, 1986, WMS.
35. AP, "Ryan Travels to New York Monday," *Kokomo Tribune*, n.d. [likely February 14 or 15, 1986].
36. "Recommended Interim Implementation of Guidelines for Hemophiliac with

AIDS/ARC Attending Middle School or High School," Western School Corporation, February 17, 1986, WMS.

37. Colby, interview, RWOHP.
38. "Recommended Interim Implementation of Guidelines," WMS. See also Christopher M. MacNeil, "Ryan Poses No Threat," *Kokomo Tribune*, February 14, 1986, n.p.
39. "Journalists Barred Friday at Western," *Kokomo Tribune*, February 18, 1986.
40. "Just Who Was Covering Whom?," *Indianapolis Star*, February 23, 1986, 6B.
41. *NBC Nightly News*, February 21, 1986, record no. 548480, VTNA.
42. *CBS Evening News*, February 21, 1986, record no. 308411, VTNA.
43. *CBS Evening News*, February 21, 1986, VTNA.
44. ABC, *World News Tonight*, February 21, 1986, record no. 101074, VTNA.
45. ABC, *World News Tonight*, February 20, 1986, record no. 101064, VTNA.
46. Christopher M. MacNeil, "Western Absentees above 40%," *Kokomo Tribune*, February 21, 1986, 1; *NBC Nightly News*, February 21, 1986, VTNA.
47. *NBC Nightly News*, February 21, 1986, VTNA.
48. *Scott Bogart v. Ryan White*, Howard County Circuit Court, State of Indiana, cause no. 49192, filed February 21, 1986, WMS.
49. "Many Hear Decision," *Kokomo Tribune*, February 22, 1986.
50. ABC, *World News Tonight*, February 21, 1986, VTNA.
51. *NBC Nightly News*, February 21, 1986, VTNA.
52. Christopher M. MacNeil, "White Says Benefit Could Be Starting Point," *Kokomo Tribune*, March 23, 1986, 6; Rogers Worthington, article draft, February 26, 1986, WMS, later revised and published as Rogers Worthington, "Kokomo Bristles over Publicity on AIDS Boy's Plight," *Chicago Tribune*, March 4, 1986, 4.
53. Patton, *Fatal Advice*.
54. Mike Hippler to "Student Body President of Western Middle School," February 24, 1986, WMS.
55. Jeff L. Hayward, letter to the editor, *Kokomo Tribune*, February 27, 1986, 5.
56. "AIDS in Queens and Kokomo," *New York Times*, February 27, 1986, A22.
57. AP, "Kokomo Wants to Better Image with AIDS Research Fund Drive," *Indianapolis Star*, March 17, 1986, 29.
58. Lawson, interview, RWOHP.
59. AP, "Kokomo Wants to Better Image with AIDS Research Fund Drive."
60. MacNeil, "White Says Benefit Could Be Starting Point." See also Bob Garrison, "AIDS Campaign Suggested Here," *Kokomo Tribune*, April 13, 1986, 17.
61. Bagby, interview, RWOHP; AP, "Group Ends Fight against AIDS Teen," *Chicago Tribune*, July 19, 1986, 6; *NBC Nightly News*, July 18, 1986, record no. 551083, VTNA.
62. *CBS Evening News*, April 22, 1986, record no. 309348, VTNA.
63. Mark Nichols, "Ryan Drops Trip, Starts to School," *Indianapolis Star*, April 11, 1986, 1.
64. AP, "US Diving Indoor Championships: Louganis' Gold Medal Goes to 14-Year-Old

Boy," *Los Angeles Times*, April 21, 1986, www.latimes.com/archives/la-xpm-1986-04-21-sp-849-story.html; John Shaughnessy, "Diver Gives Lesson in Friendship," *Indianapolis Star*, August 19, 1987, 1B.

65. ABC, *Good Morning America*, April 19, 1986, Library 147, GR00464029, WSJV, https://media.dlib.indiana.edu/media_objects/nc5817493.
66. Michele Cohen, "AIDS Boy Fights to Be Ordinary," *Sun Sentinel* (FL), June 22, 1986, 1A; contact sheet, "To Care Is to Cure at Javits Center," April 29, 1986, Andy Warhol Photography Collection, Stanford Digital Repository, Stanford University Libraries, Stanford, CA, exhibits.stanford.edu/warhol; Michael Gross, "Fashion Industry Turns Out in Force for AIDS Benefit," *New York Times*, April 30, 1986, C1.
67. Woodrow A. Myers Jr. to Mark Lubbers, February 11, 1987, Bush for President (1987–88), box 19, L. Keith Bulen Collection, Institute for Civic Leadership and Digital Mayoral Archives, University of Indianapolis, IN. This document can also be found in folder 2: Memos from Woodrow A. Myers (~1987), Woodrow A. Myers Correspondence (1985–90), Commissioners Correspondence, Commissioners Files, Indiana State Board of Health, Indiana State Archives, Indianapolis.
68. Mark Lubbers to Mitch Daniels, February 25, 1987, Bush for President (1987–88), box 19, L. Keith Bulen Collection, Institute for Civic Leadership and Digital Mayoral Archives, University of Indianapolis, IN.
69. Handwritten notes, case conference, September 19, 1985, WMS.
70. ABC, *World News Tonight*, August 25, 1986, record no. 104511, VTNA; *CBS Evening News*, August 25, 1986, record no. 311723, VTNA. For Ryan's stints in the hospital, see "Ryan White, 14, Back in Hospital," *Kokomo Tribune*, September 17, 1986, 2; "Ryan White in Hospital," *Kokomo Tribune*, November 9, 1986, 3.
71. "24 Hours in the Crisis That Is Breaking America's Heart," *People*, August 3, 1987; "Ryan White on *People* Cover," *Indianapolis Star*, July 26, 1987, 1C; White and Cunningham, *Ryan White*.
72. *NBC Nightly News*, August 31, 1987, record no. 558073, VTNA.
73. "Indiana Student Has Smooth Transition," *Washington Post*, August 30, 1987, A11.
74. *NBC Nightly News*, August 31, 1987, VTNA.
75. AP, "Schools Bolster AIDS Curriculums," *New York Times*, September 10, 1987, B11.
76. "AIDS Victim Honored," *Orlando Sentinel*, December 21, 1987, A2.
77. ABC, *World News Tonight*, December 18, 1987, record no. 107001, VTNA.
78. Ryan White, testimony before the Presidential Commission on the HIV Epidemic, March 3, 1988, https://en.wikisource.org/wiki/Ryan_White%27s_Testimony_before_the_President%27s_Commission_on_AIDS.
79. "Teen Asks for AIDS Education," *Pensacola (FL) News Journal*, July 5, 1988, 3.
80. *I Have AIDS: A Teenager's Story*.

Chapter Four

1. Woodrow A. Myers Jr. to Mark Lubbers, February 11, 1987, Bush for President (1987–88), box 19, L. Keith Bulen Collection, Institute for Civic Leadership and Digital Mayoral Archives, University of Indianapolis, IN.
2. See, for example, Cooper, *Family Values*.
3. Hubbs, *Rednecks, Queers, and Country Music*, 6, 45 (emphasis in original). See also Vaid, *Virtual Equality*.
4. Gomer, *White Balance*, 157.
5. John J. O'Connor, "Review/Television; AIDS and Hemophilia," *New York Times*, January 16, 1989; Vaid, *Virtual Equality*.
6. *NBC Nightly News*, August 31, 1988, record no. 564089, VTNA; Jeff Kunerth, "Wooing the Filmmakers: Small Town Reaches for Film Fame, Fortune as Tinseltown South," *Orlando Sentinel*, December 23, 1990, www.orlandosentinel.com/news/os-xpm-1990-12-23-9012230234-story.html.
7. Patton, *Fatal Advice*.
8. The quotation in the subheading comes from a 2011 oral history interview with Western School Corporation nurse Bev Ashcraft, who relayed an anecdote about meeting a woman from Cincinnati during her spring break vacation to Fort Myers, Florida. Upon learning that Ashcraft hailed from Kokomo, the Cincinnatian reportedly replied, "You're from that horrible town where they're mistreating this child with AIDS." Ashcraft, interview, RWOHP. Michael Specter, "AIDS Victim's Right to Attend Public School Tested in Corn Belt," *Washington Post*, September 3, 1985, www.washingtonpost.com/archive/politics/1985/09/03/aids-victims-right-to-attend-public-school-tested-in-corn-belt/8ffb6ac0-93cc-4c6f-88da-f3bb23664294/.
9. Rosemary Canter to J. O. Smith, September 10, 1985, object no. 2012.073.0005–26, HCHS.
10. Carter, interview, RWOHP; Brier, "'Save Our Kids, Keep AIDS Out.'"
11. Hubbs, *Rednecks, Queers, and Country Music*; Cram, "(Dis)locating Queer Citizenship."
12. David C. Lohse, letter to the editor, *Kokomo Tribune*, March 6, 1986, 7; Lassiter and Crespino, *Myth of Southern Exceptionalism*.
13. Jeff L. Hayward, letter to the editor, *Kokomo Tribune*, February 27, 1986, 5.
14. Lawson, interview, RWOHP.
15. Stephen J. Daily, letter to the editor, *Fort Wayne (IN) News Sentinel*, September 1987 (no specific date), WMS.
16. Bilodeau, interview, RWOHP.
17. Wiles, interview, RWOHP.
18. See, for instance, Casey Patrick, "Hamilton County Begins to Reconcile a Shameful Klan Past," *Indianapolis Monthly*, June 11, 2020, indianapolismonthly.com/longform/hamilton-county-begins-to-reconcile-a-shameful-klan-past. See also Egan, *Fever in the Heartland*; Gordon, *Second Coming of the KKK*; Madison, *Ku Klux Klan in the Heartland*; and Moore, *Citizen Klansmen*.

19. Bilodeau, interview, RWOHP.
20. *NBC Nightly News*, August 31, 1988, VTNA.
21. Steve Hall, "Film Shows Ryan White's Struggle for Understanding," *Indianapolis Star*, December 18, 1988, A1.
22. Dave Wiethop, "ABC Network Promises Accurate Portrait of Area," *Kokomo Tribune*, January 15, 1989, 2.
23. Mary Hatwood Futrell and Don Cameron to state presidents, state executive directors, and local presidents of the National Education Association, January 2, 1989, WMS.
24. KIDSNET, study guide on *The Ryan White Story*, January 1989, WMS. See also ABC, *World News Tonight*, n.d., Library 290, GR00464273, WSJV, https://media.dlib.indiana.edu/media_objects/cj82kt285.
25. *The Ryan White Story* was directed by John Herzfeld and aired on ABC. The quotes and descriptions in the following few paragraphs come from this TV film.
26. "KT streettalk [*sic*]: Did You Watch 'The Ryan White Story' Last Week?," *Kokomo Tribune*, January 23, 1989.
27. Gomer, *White Balance*, 157.
28. Robert Sargent, response to *The Ryan White Story*, February 1, 1989, object no. 2011.012.0004-3a–5m, Ryan White Collection, HCHS.
29. Susan Sandberg, letter to the editor, *Kokomo Tribune*, January 20, 1989.
30. Sargent, response to *The Ryan White Story*, HCHS.
31. Scott L. Miley, "Ryan White Film Flops in Kokomo," *Indianapolis Star*, January 18, 1989, C1.
32. Ken Armstrong, letter to the editor, *Indianapolis Star*, January 29, 1989, F3.
33. Steve Alley, letter to the editor, *Indianapolis Star*, January 21, 1989, A16.
34. Amy Royal, letter to the editor, *Kokomo Tribune*, January 20, 1989. See also Dave Wiethop, "Teens Debunk 'Ryan White Story,'" *Kokomo Tribune*, February 18, 1989, 1.
35. Ron Colby, "Press Release regarding *The Ryan White Story*," January 17, 1989, WMS.
36. Mildred K. Staples to Ron Colby, April 12, 1990, WMS.
37. J. Z., unpublished letter to the editor, *Kokomo Tribune*, postmarked April 12, 1990, object no. 2011.012.0001-5, HCHS.
38. Pamela Palmer, unpublished letter to the editor, *Kokomo Tribune*, April 10, 1990, object no. 2011.012.0001-1, HCHS; Ferries, interview, RWOHP.
39. *CBS Evening News*, April 9, 1990, record no. 332606, VTNA.
40. Bagby, interview, RWOHP.
41. Rosselot, interview, RWOHP.
42. Genovese, interview, RWOHP.
43. See, for one, Marsha Rouse, letter to the editor, *Kokomo Tribune*, March 13, 1986, 7. "I am ashamed to say that I am a citizen of this 'fair' city of Kokomo," the letter began. Rouse also compared her fellow townspeople to "a Grade-B Western showing a lynch mob scene."

44. Justin McCarthy, "Gallup Vault: Fear and Anxiety during the 1980s AIDS Crisis," Gallup, June 28, 2019, news.gallup.com/vault/259643/gallup-vault-fear-anxiety-during-1980s-AIDS-crisis.aspx.
45. Patrick Curry, letter to the editor, *Kokomo Tribune*, April 19, 1990, 6.

Chapter Five

1. AP, "Ryan White's Former Foes Rally for Him," *Sun Sentinel*, April 5, 1990, 3A.
2. Watney, *Policing Desire*, 7.
3. Jane Gross, "Funerals for AIDS Victims," *New York Times*, February 13, 1987, B1.
4. Ashcraft, interview, RWOHP.
5. Jeff Swiatek, "Ryan's Death Becomes Media Event," *Indianapolis Star*, April 9, 1990, A9; Joan Hanauer, "New 'Wings' a Winner; NBC Still on Top," *Indianapolis Star*, April 25, 1990, B16; *NBC Nightly News*, August 16, 1985, record no. 545304, VTNA.
6. "Despite His Trials, Ryan Spoke Out for AIDS Kids," *Indianapolis Star*, April 9, 1990, A8; AP, "AIDS Victim Ryan White Losing Battle with Disease," *Daily Times* (Salisbury, MD), April 3, 1990, 28; George Stuteville, "Celebrities Rally around Ryan," *Indianapolis Star*, April 4, 1990, A1.
7. Stuteville, "Celebrities Rally around Ryan."
8. AP, "AIDS Victim Ryan White Losing Battle with Disease"; Stuteville, "Celebrities Rally around Ryan."
9. "Ryan White, Whose AIDS Story Moved the World, Is Near Death," *Los Angeles Times*, April 2, 1990 (afternoon edition), 1; ABC, *World News Tonight*, April 2, 1990, record no. 128058, VTNA; *CBS Evening News*, April 2, 1990, record no. 332324, VTNA; *NBC Nightly News*, April 2, 1990, record no. 574500, VTNA.
10. See AP, "Ryan White's AIDS Battle Nears Its End," *Orlando Sentinel*, April 3, 1990, A1.
11. George Papajohn, "Ryan White's Struggle to Live Moves a Nation," *Chicago Tribune*, April 4, 1990, D1.
12. *NBC Nightly News*, April 4, 1990, record no. 574761, VTNA.
13. AP, "Ryan White's AIDS Battle Nears Its End."
14. ABC, *Nightline*, "The Best of *Nightline*" (clip show), April 24, 1990, record no. 646698, VTNA.
15. Jack Friedman with Bill Shaw, "Amazing Grace: The Quiet Victories of Ryan White," *People*, May 30, 1988, 88.
16. Judy Keen and Desda Moss, "Ryan Inspired Dignity for All AIDS Patients," *USA Today*, April 3, 1990, 1A.
17. "The Shining Spirit of Ryan White," *Chicago Tribune*, April 4, 1990, N18.
18. *NBC Nightly News*, April 4, 1990, VTNA.
19. *A Current Affair* (nationally syndicated television program), April 3, 1990, Library 371, GR00464346, WSJV, https://media.dlib.indiana.edu/media_objects/2514p574b.

20. Malcolm Gladwell, "President Calls for End to AIDS Discrimination," *Washington Post*, March 30, 1990, www.washingtonpost.com/archive/politics/1990/03/30/president-calls-for-end-to-aids-discrimination/60890a52-cae2-4b24-969a-df7c884118dd/; Rob Stein, "Bush Pledges 'To Fight Like Hell' against AIDS," UPI, March 29, 1990, www.upi.com/Archives/1990/03/29/Bush-pledges-to-fight-like-hell-against-AIDS/4111638686800/.
21. George H. W. Bush, "Remarks at a Tree-Planting Ceremony in Indianapolis, Indiana," April 3, 1990, George H. W. Bush Presidential Library and Museum, College Station, TX, https://bush41library.tamu.edu/archives/public-papers/1716; Dorothy Petroskey, "A Time to Plant, a Time to Speak," *Indianapolis Star*, April 4, 1990, A1. Bush, who in his 1988 campaign had vowed to focus on environmental concerns, also used the tree-planting ceremony to implore the US Senate to pass the Clean Air Act. He succeeded in this respect, as the bill passed by an overwhelming margin. See Fleegler, *Brutal Campaign*.
22. "'Let It Be Ryan's Tree,'" *Indianapolis Star*, April 4, 1990, A1.
23. Edna Gundersen, "Mellencamp Visits Ryan White," *USA Today*, April 6, 1990, 2D.
24. AP, "President Visits Bedridden Teen," *Clarksville (TN) Leaf-Chronicle*, April 4, 1990, 10A; Bush, "Remarks at a Tree-Planting Ceremony in Indianapolis, Indiana."
25. "Ryan Wasn't There, But His Presence Was Felt," *Indianapolis Star*, April 8, 1990, A14; Reverend Jesse Jackson, remarks at Farm Aid, April 7, 1990, uploaded to YouTube on June 21, 2012, www.youtube.com/watch?v=5FSgUZCrtGU.
26. John, *Love Is the Cure*, 20; AP, "Elton Gives Patients Gifts, Visits Ryan," *Indianapolis Star*, April 6, 1990, A15.
27. Jeanne White, interview by Sarah Purcell, *Home* (daytime TV show), in Library 368, GR00464343, WSJV, https://media.dlib.indiana.edu/media_objects/wm118910v. *People* had secured the exclusive rights to cover Ryan's final illness and death. See Beverly K. Bell, "Jeanne White Remembers," *Indianapolis Monthly*, June 1990, 83; Linda Gillis, "Magazine Captures Ryan's Last Days," *Indianapolis News*, April 18, 1990, B1; Bob Sipchen, "Eastern European Upheaval Brings Focus on Castro," *Los Angeles Times*, May 24, 1990, E16; "The Last Days of Ryan White," *People*, April 23, 1990.
28. John, *Love Is the Cure*, 21.
29. Mike Redmond, "Farewell to Farm Aid," *Indianapolis News*, April 9, 1990, B1.
30. UPI, "President, Others Exress [*sic*] Sorrow over Ryan White's Death," April 9, 1990, www.upi.com/Archives/1990/04/09/President-others-exress-sorrow-over-Ryan-Whites-death/5990639633600/.
31. Thomas B. Rosenstiel, "Hostages' Release Grabs Public's Interest," *Los Angeles Times*, May 10, 1990, A28.
32. *A Current Affair*, April 3, 1990, WSJV; Reverend Ray "Bud" Probasco used this same formulation ("a disease, not a dirty word") in his eulogy for Ryan. See Joan Todd, "Ryan White 'Humanitized' AIDS," UPI, April 11, 1990, www.upi.com/Archives/1990/04/11/Ryan-White-humanitized-AIDS/7339639806400/.

33. "AIDS Claims Ryan White after Five-Year Battle," *ISBH Bulletin*, April 1990, 14, object no. 2011.012.0012, Ryan White Collection, HCHS.
34. Virginia B. Wohlgemuth, letter to the editor, *Indianapolis Star*, April 18, 1990, A21.
35. August C. Barnes, letter to the editor, *Indianapolis Star*, April 18, 1990, A21.
36. "AIDS Claims Ryan White after Five-Year Battle," HCHS.
37. Jay B. Shaw to Ron Colby, April 9, 1990, WMS.
38. M. Vic Reiling to Ron Colby, April 13, 1990, WMS.
39. Brent Larkin, "Kokomo Can Breathe Now, Ryan's Dead," *Cleveland Plain Dealer*, n.d. [April 1990], WMS.
40. "'Innocent Victim' Ryan White Dies," *New Works News* (Indianapolis) 9, no. 8 (May 1990): 5, series 1: Periodicals, HQ 75.W62, M 1242, Michael Bohr Collection, Indy Pride Chris Gonzalez Library and Archives (ca. 1960s–2016), Manuscript and Visual Collections Department, William Henry Smith Memorial Library, IHS.
41. Greg McDaniel, letter to the editor, *New Works News* 9, no. 8 (May 1990): 3, Bohr Collection, IHS.
42. Ronald Reagan, "'We Owe It to Ryan,'" *Washington Post*, April 11, 1990, www.washingtonpost.com/archive/opinions/1990/04/11/we-owe-it-to-ryan/5d132882-b7e5-48dc-950c-e91003f1a690/.
43. ABC, *Nightline*, April 11, 1990, record no. 64687, VTNA.
44. Debbie Howlett, "Activists Warn Fight Is Far from Over," *USA Today*, April 12, 1990, 1A.
45. Eric Lichtblau, "Reagan Rejects Federal AIDS Anti-Bias Law," *Los Angeles Times*, August 3, 1988, www.latimes.com/archives/la-xpm-1988-08-03-mn-6748-story.html.
46. Dave Walter, "Straights Leading Gays," *The Advocate*, May 22, 1990, 29.
47. For more examples of the "turning point" framing, see "AIDS Claims Ryan White after Five-Year Battle," HCHS; ABC, *Nightline*, April 11, 1990, VTNA.
48. Reagan, "'We Owe It to Ryan.'"
49. Vic Caleca, "Service at Second Presbyterian Expected to Draw Hundreds," *Indianapolis Star*, April 11, 1990, A1.
50. Vic Caleca, "Ryan's Funeral to Be Open for the Public He Inspired," *Indianapolis Star*, April 10, 1990, A14.
51. *CBS Evening News*, April 11, 1990, record no. 332161, VTNA; Bruce C. Smith, "Spirit Warmed Mourners Forced to Wait Outside," *Indianapolis Star*, April 12, 1990, A1; White with Dworkin, *Weeding Out the Tears*, 9–10.
52. Rosselot, interview, RWOHP.
53. Seating chart, Ryan White funeral service, Attend Funeral of Ryan White—4/11/90, Indianapolis, Indiana (OA/ID 01905), Ann Brock files, Office of the First Lady—Scheduling, George H. W. Bush Presidential Records: Staff and Office Files, George H. W. Bush Presidential Library and Museum, College Station, TX.
54. *NBC Nightly News*, April 8, 1990, record no. 574838, VTNA.

55. White with Dworkin, *Weeding Out the Tears*, 5–6.
56. Beverly Beyette, "Ryan, We Hardly Knew You, VIPs Mourn," *Los Angeles Times*, April 12, 1990, A20; White with Dworkin, *Weeding Out the Tears*, 6; Will Higgins, "The Unusual, Unforgettable Way Indy Buried Ryan White," *Indianapolis Star*, April 9, 2015, www.indystar.com/story/life/2015/04/09/buried-ryan-white/25424315/.
57. Probasco, interview, RWOHP, 2.
58. Program from Ryan White's funeral, April 11, 1990, Second Presbyterian Church, Indianapolis, box 13, M 1242, Bohr Collection, IHS.
59. Program from Ryan White's funeral, IHS; Jeff Zogg, "Friends and Stars to Be Pallbearers," *Indianapolis News*, April 11, 1990, A1.
60. Ken Kusmer, "Farewell to the Young Symbol of Courage," *Washington Post* (AP), April 12, 1990, C1, www.washingtonpost.com/archive/lifestyle/1990/04/12/farewell-to-the-young-symbol-of-courage/b527b412-2b33-4eb3-af65-16f738761507/; White with Dworkin, *Weeding Out the Tears*, 10. Though Rod Stewart had originally recorded and released the song—which was written by Burt Bacharach and Carole Bayer Sager—the 1985 version featuring Dionne Warwick, Gladys Knight, Stevie Wonder, and Elton John is more widely known.
61. ABC, *Nightline*, April 11, 1990, VTNA; Beyette, "Ryan, We Hardly Knew You, VIPs Mourn." For more on the "de-gaying" of AIDS, see King, *Safety in Numbers*, esp. chap. 5; Vaid, *Virtual Equality*; and Canaday, *Queer Career*, esp. chaps. 5 and 6.
62. *NBC Nightly News*, April 11, 1990, record no. 574321, VTNA.
63. John, *Love Is the Cure*, 22.
64. White with Dworkin, *Weeding Out the Tears*, 11.
65. Program from Ryan White's funeral, IHS.
66. Many thanks to Ted Frantz for his guidance on this point.
67. Todd, "Ryan White 'Humanitized' AIDS."
68. White with Dworkin, *Weeding Out the Tears*, 10, 11.
69. Howlett, "Activists Warn Fight Is Far from Over."
70. Larkin, "Kokomo Can Breathe Now, Ryan's Dead."
71. Howlett, "Activists Warn Fight Is Far from Over."
72. ABC, *Nightline*, April 11, 1990, VTNA.
73. Dan Carpenter, "His Days Were Numbered; His Friends Were Countless," *Indianapolis Star*, April 12, 1990, A16.
74. ABC, *Nightline*, April 11, 1990, VTNA.
75. Carpenter, "His Days Were Numbered."
76. ABC, *Nightline*, April 11, 1990, VTNA.
77. Dan Carpenter, "Where Was Reagan in Early Years of AIDS?," *Indianapolis Star*, April 17, 1990, D1.
78. Wojnarowicz, *Close to the Knives*, 122.
79. The Marys, Stumpf/Kane solicitation, included in *Anonymous Queer* (June 1992), from Joy Episalla's s private collection, found in Levine, "How to Do Things with Dead Bodies."

80. Episalla, interview, ACT UP Oral History Project, https://actuporalhistory.org/numerical-interviews/036-joy-episalla; Episalla, interview, March 17, 2016, *Visual Arts and the AIDS Epidemic: An Oral History Project*, www.aaa.si.edu/collections/interviews/oral-history-interview-joy-episalla-16324; Levine, "How to Do Things with Dead Bodies."
81. Episalla, interview, ACT UP Oral History Project; Episalla, interview, March 17, 2016, *Visual Arts and the AIDS Epidemic*.
82. Robinson, interview, ACT UP Oral History Project, https://actuporalhistory.org/numerical-interviews/082-david-robinson; *The Ashes Action*, dir. James Wentzy, *AIDS Community Television* (1992), available via the ACT UP Oral History Project, https://actuporalhistory.org/actions/political-funerals. The Watney quotation scrolls across the bottom of the screen in yellow. See also Bryan-Wilson, *Fray*, esp. chap. 3.

    Nino Testa complicates activist and scholarly discourses that have "reduce[d] the AIDS Quilt to a homogenous art object more or less politically equivalent to conservative and sentimental mass media representations" and positioned the quilt "as disengaged from direct-action politics." Although Testa leans on the work of Sarah Schulman, for one, he also insists that Schulman and other scholars and activists have overlooked continuities between the radical politics of ACT UP and presumably "sentimental" projects like the AIDS Memorial Quilt. See Testa, "'If You Are Reading It, I Am Dead,'" quoted on 37 and 54.
83. Episalla, interview, ACT UP Oral History Project; Episalla, interview, March 17, 2016, *Visual Arts and the AIDS Epidemic*; Mark Lowe Fisher political funeral, November 2, 1992, footage by James Wentzy, New York Public Library tape no. 1230-B, available via the ACT UP Historical Archive, https://actuporalhistory.org/actions/political-funerals. See also Dan Royles, "Love and Rage."
84. Royles, "Love and Rage."
85. Tim Bailey political funeral, July 1, 1993, footage by James Wentzy, New York Public Library tape no. 1227-AB, available via the ACT UP Oral History Project, https://actupny.org/nypl/description/01227.html.
86. As Dan Royles has shown, ACT UP Philadelphia actually "grew in numbers by seeking out new members from the city's low-income communities of color." Royles, "Love and Rage"; Royles, *To Make the Wounded Whole*.

Chapter Six

1. US Congress, Senate, Committee on Labor and Human Resources, *HIV Emergency Relief Grant Program: Report (To Accompany S. 2240)*, 101st Cong., 2d Sess., April 24 (legislative day April 18), 1990, S. Rep. 101-273.
2. AP, "Ryan White's Former Foes Rally for Him," *Sun Sentinel*, April 5, 1990, 3A.
3. Senator Jesse Helms, speaking on S. 2240, *Congressional Record* (Senate), 101st Cong., 2d Sess., May 14, 1990, 10249, 10251.
4. Helms, speaking on S. 2240, *Congressional Record*, May 14, 1990, 10246, 10249.

5. For "a politically safe symbol," see Susan F. Rasky, "How the Politics Shifted on AIDS Funds," *New York Times*, May 20, 1990, 22. For "hierarchy of victimhood," see Petro, *After the Wrath of God*, 2.
6. "Senators Say 'Wait' . . . While AIDS Kills Philadelphians," *Philadelphia Daily News*, September 20, 1990, box 121, folder 14 (legislation: Ryan White CARE Act of 1990), NGLTF. For the proposed Ryan White Amendment, see Senator Jesse Helms, statement on S. 2240, *Congressional Record* (Senate), 101st Cong., 2d Sess., May 16, 1990, 10698; and Donovan, "Problem with Making AIDS Comfortable," 131.
7. Senator Ted Kennedy, statement on S. 2240, *Congressional Record* (Senate), 101st Cong., 2d Sess., March 6, 1990, 3530.
8. National Organizations Responding to AIDS, "Over Fifty National Organizations Call for AIDS Care Response," press release, March 5, 1990, included in US Congress, House of Representatives, Committee on the Budget, *AIDS Funding Issues—Impact Aid, Early Intervention, Research, and Prevention: Hearing before the Task Force on Human Resources*, 101st Cong., 2d Sess., March 7, 1990, 110. Hurricane Hugo devastated parts of the Caribbean—including the US Virgin Islands and Puerto Rico—before hitting Georgia, the Carolinas, and Virginia in September 1989.
9. ACT UP flyer, "A NATURAL DISASTER IS STORMING THE NATION!," n.d. [likely fall 1990], box 121, folder 14, NGLTF.
10. Kitzinger and Peel, "De-gaying and Re-gaying of AIDS," 177; Vaid, *Virtual Equality*, esp. chap. 3. As Jih-Fei Cheng, Alexandra Juhasz, and Nishant Shahani put it,

> One of the primary orientations of the earliest segments of the AIDS crisis was a go-to analysis, and its associated set of procedures, policies, and politics, that insisted on the disarticulation of disease or infection from identity. At the time, and moving forward across the crises, this became a fundamental orientation and response to the bigoted and scientifically unsound underpinnings and ongoing manifestations of the epidemic where stigma was the [undeserved] outcome for entire classes of humans, producing immense violence and oceans of bad information in one stupid, lasting swipe (initially about and against homosexuals, heroin users, hemophiliacs, and Haitians but eventually and quickly crystallizing and sticking to gay men). The earlier activist credo—AIDS is not about who you are but what you do—armed people to better understand that safer sex practices, attempts at healthy living, and clean-needle use (to name a few of what you do) mattered above identity categories (Cheng, Juhasz, and Shahani, "Introduction," 18).

11. Watkins-Hayes, *Remaking a Life*, 3, 1. Also see chap. 2 of her book.
12. See Nicholas and Abrams, "Boarder Babies with AIDS in Harlem"; Andiman, "Where Have All the 'AIDS Babies' Gone?" For more on women and HIV/AIDS, see Patton, *Last Served?*; Treichler, *How to Have Theory in an Epidemic*; Hogan,

Women Take Care; O'Daniel, *Holding On*; and Watkins-Hayes, *Remaking a Life*. Many thanks to Sarah Schulman for her guidance on this point.

13. Eric Rofes, "Gay Lib vs. AIDS: Averting Civil War in the 1990s," *Out/Look* 8 (Spring 1990): 8–17.
14. Michael Callen, "AIDS Is a Gay Disease," *PWA Coalition Newsline* 42 (March 1989), found in King, *Safety in Numbers*, 169.
15. Siplon, *AIDS and the Policy Struggle in the United States*, 95.
16. Theorist Jack Halberstam coined the term "metronormativity" to critique the scholarly tendency to focus on queer life in urban spaces. Scott Herring and others have built upon Halberstam's insights through their explorations of queer life in rural environments. See especially Howard, *Men Like That*; E. Johnson, *Sweet Tea*; Herring, *Another Country*; C. Johnson, *Just Queer Folks*; Manalansan et al., "Queering the Middle"; and Gray, Johnson, and Gilley, *Queering the Countryside.*
17. Senator Lloyd Bentsen, statement on S. 2240, *Congressional Record* (Senate), 101st Cong., 2d Sess., March 6, 1990, 3545.
18. For the urban core as a source of anxiety in late twentieth-century American political culture, see Macek, *Urban Nightmares*.
19. See especially the July 1985 cover of *Life* magazine, which cautioned, "Now No One Is Safe from AIDS." For analysis of this cover and the historical moment in which it appeared, see Sturken, *Tangled Memories*, 151–52.
20. Senator Pete Wilson, statement on S. 2240, *Congressional Record* (Senate), 101st Cong., 2d Sess., March 6, 1990, 3546.
21. Robert Z. Alpern, Robert Brooks, Irwin M. Blank, Jay Lintner, Melva B. Jimerson, Mary A. Cooper, Ruth Flowers, and Elenora Giddings Ivory to Edward M. Kennedy, March 1, 1990, box 121, folder 14, NGLTF.
22. Mitchell Locin, "Senate OKs New AIDS Funds," *Chicago Tribune*, May 17, 1990, D1; C. W. Henderson, "Proposal for Emergency AIDS Funds for Major Cities," *AIDS Weekly*, March 19, 1990, A6–A7.
23. Elizabeth Taylor, statement on S. 2240, *Congressional Record* (Senate), 101st Cong., 2d Sess., March 6, 1990, 3538.
24. For more on austerity in the 1980s and 1990s, see Meeropol, *Surrender*; and Lichtenstein and Stein, *Fabulous Failure*. For more on the ways in which policymakers and activists used celebrities, bipartisanship, coalitional politics, atypical cases (like that of Ryan White), and the rhetoric of "disaster" and "emergency" to pass the CARE Act, see Poindexter, "Promises in the Plague."
25. Senate, Committee on Labor and Human Resources, *HIV Emergency Relief Grant Program: Report (To Accompany S. 2240)*.
26. For the rise of ACT UP, see Gould, *Moving Politics*; Carroll, *Mobilizing New York*; and Schulman, *Let the Record Show*.
27. For "sanitizing," see Rofes, "Gay Lib vs. AIDS." See also Sheridan, *Helping the Good Do Better.*
28. Rasky, "How the Politics Shifted on AIDS Funds." Very few AIDS activists spoke

out against naming the CARE Act after Ryan White. One notable exception was former congressperson and Democratic vice presidential nominee Geraldine Ferraro. During her keynote address at the Human Rights Campaign Fund's New England Dinner in the fall of 1990, Ferraro "attacked her former colleagues in Congress for naming the AIDS care bill after Ryan White," the *Gay Community News* reported. Gordon Gottlieb, "HRCF Holds Annual Dinner," *Gay Community News* (Boston), November 2, 1990, 3.

29. Helms, speaking on S. 2240, *Congressional Record* (Senate), May 14, 1990, 10249, 10248.
30. Helms, speaking on S. 2240, *Congressional Record* (Senate), 101st Cong., 2d Sess., May 15, 1990, 10329; Helms, speaking on S. 2240, *Congressional Record* (Senate), May 14, 1990, 10249.
31. Helms, speaking on S. 2240, *Congressional Record* (Senate), May 14, 1990, 10249.
32. Helms, speaking on S. 2240, *Congressional Record* (Senate), May 14, 1990, 10249.
33. Tony Snow, "Ryan White's 'Legacy,'" *Washington Times*, April 13, 1990, n.p., box 1170, folder 7a, Record Group 2, Senatorial Papers, Legislative Files (1972–2002), Jesse Helms Papers, JHCA.
34. James P. Paget, letter to the editor, *Human Events*, May 26, 1990, 22.
35. Helms, speaking on S. 2240, *Congressional Record* (Senate), May 14, 1990, 10248.
36. Jesse Helms to Orrin Hatch, May 9, 1990, box 1170, folder 7b, JHCA.
37. Helms, speaking on S. 2240, *Congressional Record* (Senate), May 14, 1990, 10249.
38. Helms, speaking on S. 2240, *Congressional Record* (Senate), May 14, 1990, 10249.
39. Helms, speaking on S. 2240, *Congressional Record* (Senate), May 14, 1990, 10249.
40. Senator Gordon Humphrey, speaking on S. 2240, *Congressional Record* (Senate), 101st Cong., 2d Sess., May 16, 1990, 10712.
41. Fumento, *Myth of Heterosexual AIDS*, 331.
42. Fumento, *Myth of Heterosexual AIDS*, 328.
43. Dick Thompson, "The AIDS Political Machine," *Time*, January 22, 1990, https://content.time.com/time/subscriber/article/0,33009,969229,00.html.
44. Helms, speaking on S. 2240, *Congressional Record* (Senate), May 14, 1990, 10251–52.
45. Murphy, "No Time for an AIDS Backlash," 8 (emphasis in original).
46. Ronald Bayer, "The AIDS Plague and the Body Politic," *Washington Post*, January 21, 1990, www.washingtonpost.com/archive/entertainment/books/1990/01/21/the-aids-plague-and-the-body-politic/182029d0-71ec-4cbb-90e1-a119228fdc15/.
47. Jonathan Bell, "Between Private and Public," 180. See also Schulman, *Let the Record Show*.
48. Helms to Hatch, May 9, 1990, box 1170, folder 7b, JHCA.
49. Comprehensive AIDS Resources Emergency Act, S. 2240, 101st Cong., 104 Stat. 576, introduced March 6, 1990. For the relevant section concerning the allocation of Title II funds to "infants, children, women, and families," see Title II, "HIV Care Grants," section 2541. This became section 2612 (42 USC 300ff-22) in the final version of the law.
50. Helms, speaking on S. 2240, *Congressional Record* (Senate), May 14, 1990, 10250.

Through the passage of Senate Amendment 1630, this waiver was removed from the final version of the bill.

51. Helms, speaking on S. 2240, *Congressional Record* (Senate), May 14, 1990, 10251.
52. Senator Orrin Hatch, speaking on S. 2240, *Congressional Record* (Senate), 101st Cong., 2d Sess., May 14, 1990, 10244.
53. Senator Dan Coats, speaking on S. 2240, *Congressional Record* (Senate), 101st Cong., 2d Sess., May 16, 1990, 10715.
54. Rasky, "How the Politics Shifted on AIDS Funds."
55. Davidson, *Concerto for the Left Hand*, 50.
56. Sheridan, *Helping the Good Do Better.*
57. Rasky, "How the Politics Shifted on AIDS Funds."
58. Donovan, "Problem with Making AIDS Comfortable"; *Congressional Record* (Senate), 101st Cong., 2d Sess., May 16, 1990.
59. Matt Fisher, "A History of the Ban on Federal Funding for Syringe Exchange Programs," Center for Strategic and International Studies blog, February 7, 2012, www.csis.org/blogs/smart-global-health/history-ban-federal-funding-syringe-exchange-programs.
60. Harsono et al., "Criminalization of HIV Exposure," 3.
61. For "HIV monsters," see Tomso, "HIV Monsters."
62. Hoppe, *Punishing Disease*, 114–15.
63. Hoppe, *Punishing Disease*, 122.
64. George H. W. Bush, "Statement of Administration Policy: H.R. 4785—AIDS Prevention Act of 1990," May 24, 1990, APP, www.presidency.ucsb.edu/documents/statement-administration-policy-hr-4785-aids-prevention-act-1990. Because the Senate bill (S. 2240)—which had passed several days before Bush made this statement—also focused on HIV/AIDS, the administration's critique could apply to that bill, as well. For more on the reconciliation process, see Abramson, "Rules of Engagement," esp. chap. 5.
65. C. W. Henderson, "Bush Signs AIDS Bill," *AIDS Weekly*, August 27, 1990, A1.
66. For more on devolution and the CARE Act, see Siplon, "Washington's Response to the AIDS Epidemic."
67. Royles, "HIV/AIDS in the United States." See also Siplon, "Washington's Response to the AIDS Epidemic," 803.

Chapter Seven

1. White with Dworkin, *Weeding Out the Tears*, 188, 189; Douglas A. Levy, "AIDS Activists March on Washington," UPI, September 30, 1991; Episalla, interview, February 23, 2016, *Visual Arts and the AIDS Epidemic: An Oral History Project*, www.aaa.si.edu/collections/interviews/oral-history-interview-joy-episalla-16324. According to ACT UP New York's website, eighty-four people were arrested during this protest. See ACT UP Historical Archive, "ACT UP/NY Chronology 1991," https://actupny.org/documents/cron-91.html, accessed November 12, 2023.

2. Geraldine A. Collier, "Health Officials Mourn Cuts in AIDS Funding," *Telegram & Gazette* (MA), September 14, 1990, 3.
3. Philip J. Hilts, "Panel Approves Large Cut in AIDS Relief Bill," *New York Times*, October 24, 1990, A20.
4. Siplon, "Washington's Response to the AIDS Epidemic."
5. Sheryl Gay Stolberg, "Clinton Decides Not to Finance Needle Program," *New York Times*, April 21, 1998, A1. My thanks go to one of the external reviewers for suggesting this article.
6. Mark Schoofs and Rachel Zimmerman, "Clinton Says He Regrets Decision against Needle-Exchange Program," *Wall Street Journal*, July 12, 2002, www.wsj .com/articles/SB1026437756184060600.
7. Andrew Sullivan, "When Plagues End: Notes on the Twilight of an Epidemic," *New York Times Magazine*, November 10, 1996.
8. Warner, *Trouble with Normal*, 197.
9. ABC, *World News Tonight*, October 15, 1990, record no. 125297, VTNA.
10. ABC, *World News Tonight*, October 15, 1990, VTNA.
11. Sandra Jacobs, "AIDS System in Peril," *Sun Sentinel*, September 24, 1990, 1B.
12. Gerald S. Cohen, "Senate Panel Guts AIDS Spending Bill," *Telegram & Gazette*, September 13, 1990, A6.
13. AP, "AIDS Victim's Mom Decries Bill," *Chicago Tribune*, September 27, 1990, 3.
14. Elizabeth Mann, "Protesters Act Up for AIDS Funds," *Seattle Times*, October 7, 1990, B2; "AIDS Cuts Protested," *Los Angeles Sentinel*, October 11, 1990, A21; "Plan to Cut AIDS Funding Protested," *Star Tribune* (MN), October 7, 1990, 6B.
15. Memorandum, Paul Feldman to ACT UP Network, September 27, 1990, re: "OCTOBER 6—DEMAND FULL FUNDING OF FEDERAL AIDS CARE BILL," box 121, folder 14, NGLTF.
16. Von Eschen, *Paradoxes of Nostalgia*, 27.
17. ACT UP flyer, "A NATURAL DISASTER IS STORMING THE NATION!," n.d. [likely fall 1990], box 121, folder 14, NGLTF.
18. Feldman to ACT UP Network, September 27, 1990, NGLTF.
19. Hobson, *Lavender and Red*, esp. chap. 6.
20. Art Agnos and David Dinkins, "Mayors' Pleas for Help in War on AIDS," *San Francisco Chronicle*, September 12, 1990, A19, box 121, folder 14, NGLTF.
21. Philip J. Hilts, "Senate Panel Approves a Major Cut in AIDS Relief for Cities," *New York Times*, October 11, 1990, D23.
22. ACT UP New York, "Direct Action: Target Bush," n.d. [1991], identifier no. IIP486F10, Digital Library of Nonviolent Resistance, International Institute for Peace, Rutgers University, New Brunswick, NJ, https://nonviolence.rutgers.edu /document/IIP486F10.
23. Ed Boyce, "Protest in Kennebunkport," *Gay Community News*, September 14, 1991, 1; UPI, "AIDS Protest Planned at Bush Kennebunkport Compound," August 31, 1991, www.upi.com/Archives/1991/08/31/AIDS-protest-planned-at-Bush -Kennebunkport-compound/9014683611200/.

24. Hilts, "Panel Approves Large Cut in AIDS Relief Bill"; "Actress Leads Critics of US AIDS Spending," *Los Angeles Times*, June 3, 1992, 10.
25. Garretson, *Path to Gay Rights*, 112–13.
26. Dawn Schmitz, "Assessing the Candidates," *Gay Community News*, March 8, 1992; Garretson, *Path to Gay Rights*, 113–14.
27. Schmitz, "Assessing the Candidates."
28. Anthony Salvanto and Jennifer De Pinto, "George H. W. Bush: The Public's View of Him during His Presidency," CBS News, December 4, 2018, cbsnews.com/news/george-h-w-bush-the-publics-view-of-him-during-his-presidency/. For more on Buchanan's 1992 campaign, see Hemmer, *Partisans*; Ganz, *When the Clock Broke*.
29. "A New Covenant with the American People," Democratic Party Platform, July 13, 1992, APP, www.presidency.ucsb.edu/documents/1992-democratic-party-platform.
30. Elizabeth Glaser, "Address at the 1992 Democratic National Convention," July 14, 1992, Archives of Women's Political Communication, Carrie Chapman Catt Center for Women and Politics, Iowa State University, Ames, https://awpc.cattcenter.iastate.edu/2017/03/21/address-at-the-1992-dnc-july-14-1992/.
31. Andy Towle, "Bob Hattoy's Speech to the 1992 Democratic National Convention," *Towleroad*, March 5, 2007, www.towleroad.com/2007/03/bob_hattoys_spe/.
32. William J. Clinton, "Address Accepting the Presidential Nomination at the Democratic National Convention in New York," July 16, 1992, APP, www.presidency.ucsb.edu/documents/address-accepting-the-presidential-nomination-the-democratic-national-convention-new-york.
33. George H. W. Bush, "Remarks Accepting the Presidential Nomination at the Republican National Convention in Houston," August 20, 1992, APP, www.presidency.ucsb.edu/documents/remarks-accepting-the-presidential-nomination-the-republican-national-convention-houston; Mary Fisher, "A Whisper of AIDs [*sic*]," Republican National Convention, August 19, 1992, Archives of Women's Political Communication, Carrie Chapman Catt Center for Women and Politics, Iowa State University, Ames, https://awpc.cattcenter.iastate.edu/2017/03/09/a-whisper-of-aids/.
34. "AIDS: Progress and Prospects," *Washington Post*, August 24, 1992, A16. In his address, which some scholars have identified as an opening salvo in the "culture wars," Buchanan described the DNC as a "giant masquerade ball" in which "20,000 liberals and radicals came dressed up as moderates and centrists in the greatest single exhibition of cross-dressing in American political history." See especially Hartman, *War for the Soul of America*.
35. George H. W. Bush to Phil Brady (re: Ryan White CARE Act), May 28, 1992, NLGB control no. 6013, Samuel K. Skinner files, Office of the Chief of Staff to the President, George H. W. Bush Presidential Records, George H. W. Bush Presidential Library and Museum, College Station, TX.

36. Roger Porter to George H. W. Bush (re: Ryan White CARE Act), May 28, 1992, NLGB control no. 6012, Samuel K. Skinner files, Office of the Chief of Staff to the President, George H. W. Bush Presidential Records, George H. W. Bush Presidential Library and Museum, College Station, TX.
37. Glaser, "Address at the 1992 Democratic National Convention."
38. Presidential Debate in St. Louis, October 11, 1992, APP, www.presidency.ucsb.edu/documents/presidential-debate-st-louis. On the day of the debate, ACT UP had conducted its Ashes Action in Washington, DC, throwing the cremated remains of PWAs on the White House lawn. Bush was asked about the demonstration during the debate. Charles Babington, "AIDS Activists Throw Ashes at White House," *Washington Post*, October 12, 1992, www.washingtonpost.com/archive/local/1992/10/12/aids-activists-throw-ashes-at-white-house/7a9c53e0-413f-449f-8dd1-a2804d6695ec/.
39. Ronald Brownstein, "Economic Concerns Fueled Clinton's Drive to Victory," *Los Angeles Times*, November 4, 1992, www.latimes.com/archives/la-xpm-1992-11-04-mn-1323-story.html.
40. Vanessa Williams, "Gays and Lesbians of Both Parties Are Supporting Clinton," *Philadelphia Inquirer*, October 29, 1992, A12.
41. John Gallagher and Chris Bull, "Washington's New Attitude," *The Advocate*, January 26, 1993, 34–41.
42. Gran Fury, *Sexism Rears Its Unprotected Head* (1988), Gran Fury Collection, Series I: Artwork, Manuscript and Archives Division, New York Public Library, New York City, https://digitalcollections.nypl.org/items/510d47e3-5379-a3d9-e040-e00a18064a99.
43. Gran Fury, *Women Don't Get AIDS. They Just Die from It* (1992), Gran Fury Collection, Series I: Artwork, Manuscript and Archives Division, New York Public Library, New York City, https://digitalcollections.nypl.org/items/510d47e3-5399-a3d9-e040-e00a18064a99.
44. "Impact of the Expanded AIDS Surveillance Case Definition on AIDS Case Reporting—United States, First Quarter, 1993," *Morbidity and Mortality Weekly Report* 42, no. 16 (April 30, 1993): 308–10. See also Brier, *Infectious Ideas*, esp. chap. 5.
45. Taylor-Brown, "'Women Don't Get AIDS.'" Taylor-Brown's article borrowed its title from the Gran Fury poster that urged the CDC to "expand the definition of AIDS."
46. "Marchers to Bear AIDS Quilt Panels," *Washington Post*, January 12, 1993, D3.
47. Timothy J. McNulty, "Clinton Faces Full Agenda on AIDS," *Chicago Tribune*, January 3, 1993, 19.
48. "AIDS Activists Watch President Clinton Closely," *All Things Considered* (National Public Radio), January 27, 1993.
49. Philip J. Hilts, "Clinton Picks New Director of AIDS Policy," *New York Times*, November 11, 1994, A20.
50. Michael Putzel, "Clinton Starts AIDS Prevention Push," *Boston Globe*, December 2, 1993, 3.

51. Hilts, "Clinton Picks New Director of AIDS Policy"; "Clinton and AIDS," *New Republic*, December 26, 1994, 7.
52. C. W. Henderson, "AIDS Action Council Backs Clinton Health Reform Initiative," *AIDS Weekly*, October 4, 1993, 3. See also Lichtenstein and Stein, *Fabulous Failure*.
53. Mark Miller, "Is It Good for the Gays?," *Out*, March 1995, 63; "Gingrich: Let Experts Set AIDS Funds," *Atlanta Constitution*, July 6, 1995, A7; NORA Coalition Letter on HR 1872, September 8, 1995, box 32, folder 9, National Organizations Responding to AIDS (NORA), 1987–2005, AIDS Action Foundation Records (MS 2212), Special Collections Research Center, Gelman Library, George Washington University, Washington, DC. For more on the broader political context, see Hemmer, *Partisans*.
54. US Senate, Committee on Labor and Human Resources, *Report on Ryan White Care Reauthorization Act of 1995*, report 104-25, 104th Cong., 1st Sess., April 3, 1995 (legislative day March 27, 1995).
55. Senator Ted Kennedy, speaking on S. 641, *Congressional Record* (Senate), 104th Cong., 1st Sess., March 28, 1995, 9460.
56. Katharine Q. Seelye, "Helms Puts the Brakes to a Bill Financing AIDS Treatment," *New York Times*, July 5, 1995, A12.
57. Faye Fiore, "Helms Blocks Funding for AIDS Services," *Los Angeles Times*, July 7, 1995, WA5; Seelye, "Helms Puts the Brakes to a Bill Financing AIDS Treatment."
58. Seelye, "Helms Puts the Brakes to a Bill Financing AIDS Treatment."
59. Jill Stoller, letter to the editor, *New York Times*, July 7, 1995, A24.
60. "There's Just One Way to Halt the AIDS Plague: Research," *Tallahassee Democrat*, July 11, 1995, 6A.
61. Jim Smith, letter to the editor, *New York Times*, July 9, 1995, E14.
62. Senator Jesse Helms, statement on Ryan White CARE Act, July 26, 1995, box 1170, folder 7a, Jesse Helms Papers, Record Group 2 (Senatorial Papers), Legislative Files (1972–2002), JHCA.
63. Senator Jesse Helms, general statement, "Ryan White Reauthorization Act of 1995," n.d., box 1170, folder 7a, JHCA.
64. Lisa Rhodes to Senator Jesse Helms, July 21, 1995, box 1170, folder 7a, JHCA.
65. Senate Amendment no. 1854, Ryan White CARE Reauthorization Act of 1995, *Congressional Record* (Senate), 104th Cong., 1st Sess., July 26, 1995, 10741.
66. Petro, *After the Wrath of God*, 2.
67. "ACT UP Accomplishments, 1987–2012," ACT UP New York, https://actupny.com/act-up-chronology-in-brief/, accessed November 12, 2023.
68. Abdallah Fayyad, "The LGBTQ Health Clinic That Faced a Dark Truth about the AIDS Crisis," *The Atlantic*, July 22, 2019, www.theatlantic.com/health/archive/2019/07/us-aids-policy-lingering-epidemic/594445/.
69. Sullivan, "When Plagues End," 54.
70. Warner, *Trouble with Normal*, 197.
71. President Bill Clinton, Statement on Signing the Ryan White CARE Act

Amendments of 2000, October 20, 2000, APP, www.presidency.ucsb.edu /documents/statement-signing-the-ryan-white-care-act-amendments-2000–0 (emphasis in original).

72. For the "pastness of AIDS," see especially Fink, *Forget Burial.*
73. Joelle Goldstein, "Ryan White, Who Died of AIDS at 18, Would Have Turned 50 Today," *People*, December 6, 2021, https://people.com/human-interest/ryan-white -who-died-of-aids-at-18-honored-on-what-would-have-been-his-50th-birthday/.
74. See especially Cohen, *Boundaries of Blackness*; Bost, *Evidence of Being*; and Royles, *To Make the Wounded Whole.*
75. Tim Teeman, "'We're All in This Together' Is the Dumbest Lie of the Coronavirus Pandemic," *Daily Beast*, May 7, 2020, www.thedailybeast.com/were-all-in -this-together-is-the-dumbest-lie-of-the-coronavirus-pandemic.

Epilogue

1. Andrew Sullivan, "When Plagues End: Notes on the Twilight of an Epidemic," *New York Times Magazine*, November 10, 1996.
2. Peters et al., "HIV Infection Linked to Injection Use of Oxymorphone."
3. Josh Wood, "'We Still Have Darkness': The Town Where an HIV Outbreak Occurred under Mike Pence," *The Guardian*, March 8, 2020, www.theguardian .com/us-news/2020/mar/07/mike-pence-indiana-hiv-outbreak-coronavirus.
4. AP, "Pence's Handling of 2015 HIV Outbreak Gets New Scrutiny," NBCNews .com, February 28, 2020, www.nbcnews.com/politics/white-house/pence-s -handling-2015-hiv-outbreak-gets-new-scrutiny-n1144786.
5. Ryan Trares, "Pence Used Radio Show to Build Name," *The Republic* (IN), January 18, 2017, www.therepublic.com/2017/01/18/pence-used-radio-show-to -build-name/.
6. "The Pence Agenda for the 107th Congress: A Guide to Renewing the American Dream," Mike Pence for Congress (2000), https://web.archive.org/web/20010 519165033fw_/http:/cybertext.net/pence/issues.html, accessed March 25, 2023.
7. "Pence Agenda for the 107th Congress."
8. "Pence, Opponents Square Off in Debate," *Daily Journal* (IN), September 26, 2000, 1, found in Andrew Kaczynski, "Mike Pence Defended His 'Smoking Doesn't Kill' Op-Ed in a 2000 Congressional Debate," Buzzfeed, July 20, 2016, www.buzzfeednews.com/article/andrewkaczynski/mike-pence-defended-his -smoking-doesnt-kill-op-ed-in-a-2000.
9. "When Newt and Pence Were on Opposite Sides," *The Hill*, July 13, 2016, https:// thehill.com/homenews/287525-when-newt-and-pence-were-on-opposite-sides/.
10. Will Drabold, "Here's What Mike Pence Said on LGBT Issues over the Years," *Time*, July 15, 2016, https://time.com/4406337/mike-pence-gay-rights-lgbt -religious-freedom/; Mark Memmott, "'Don't Ask, Don't Tell' Repeal Gets Critical 15th Vote," National Public Radio, May 27, 2010, www.npr.org/sections /thetwo-way/2010/05/dont_ask_dont_tell_repeal_byrd.html.
11. Shari Rudavsky and Maureen Groppe, "Gov. Pence Gets Federal OK for Medicaid

Alternative," *Indianapolis Star*, January 27, 2015, www.indystar.com/story/news/politics/2015/01/27/gov-pence-gets-federal-ok-medicaid-alternative/22396503/.

12. "Apple's Tim Cook and Other Tech CEOs Blast Indiana Religious Freedom Law," NBCNews.com, March 27, 2015, www.nbcnews.com/tech/tech-news/apples-tim-cook-other-tech-ceos-blast-indiana-religious-freedom-n331736.
13. Mike Pence, "Remarks by the Vice President at a World AIDS Day Event," November 29, 2018, APP, www.presidency.ucsb.edu/documents/remarks-the-vice-president-world-aids-day-event.
14. For "politically safe," see Susan F. Rasky, "How the Politics Shifted on AIDS Funds," *New York Times*, May 20, 1990, 22. For criticism of Pence's address, see Trent Straube, "The 'Absolute Charade' of Pence's World AIDS Day Address," *POZ*, November 30, 2018, www.poz.com/article/absolute-charade-pences-world-aids-day-address-video; and Reynaldo Leanos Jr., "Pence Criticized for Not Mentioning Gay Community in World AIDS Day Speech," NBCNews.com, November 30, 2018, www.nbcnews.com/feature/nbc-out/pence-criticized-not-mentioning-gay-community-world-aids-day-speech-n942351.
15. Warner, *Trouble with Normal*, 197.
16. Pence, "Remarks by the Vice President at a World AIDS Day Event."
17. Centers for Disease Control and Prevention, *HIV Surveillance Supplemental Report*, 7.
18. Cheng, Juhasz, and Shahani, *AIDS and the Distribution of Crises*.
19. Kathryn Macapagal, "This HIV Prevention Medicine Is for Everyone: Why Do So Few People Take It?," *STAT*, January 20, 2022, www.statnews.com/2022/01/20/this-hiv-prevention-medicine-is-for-everyone-why-do-so-few-people-take-it/; "Biomedical Racism, Queer Theory, and the Monkeypox Epidemic," *Deconstructed* podcast, interview with Joseph Osmundson, August 11, 2022, https://theintercept.com/2022/08/11/monkeypox-joseph-osmundson-virology-queer-theory/.
20. The term "Hispanic" is the designation used by the Centers for Disease Control and Prevention.
21. Centers for Disease Control and Prevention, "HIV by Group," www.cdc.gov/hiv/group/index.html, accessed October 30, 2023; Kathryn Macapagal and Darnell Motley, "Eliminating HIV in Black Communities," *Scientific American*, February 20, 019, https://blogs.scientificamerican.com/voices/eliminating-hiv-in-black-communities/.
22. Mark Mazzetti, Noah Weiland, and Sheryl Gay Stolberg, "Under Pence, Politics Regularly Seeped into the Coronavirus Task Force," *New York Times*, October 8, 2020, www.nytimes.com/2020/10/08/us/politics/pence-coronavirus-task-force.html.
23. Allie Malloy and Maegan Vazquez, "Biden Warns of Winter of 'Severe Illness and Death' for Unvaccinated Due to Omicron," CNN, December 16, 2021, www.cnn.com/2021/12/16/politics/joe-biden-warning-winter/index.html.
24. A. J. McDougall, "White House to Dissolve COVID-19 Task Force in May: Report," *Daily Beast*, March 22, 2023, www.thedailybeast.com/white-house-to-dissolve-covid-19-task-force-in-may-report.

25. Joseph Osmundson, “We Can’t Fight Monkeypox ‘Ourselves,’” *Dame*, August 25, 2022, www.damemagazine.com/2022/08/25/we-cant-fight-monkeypox-ourselves/.
26. Amna Nawaz and Dorothy Hastings, “Epidemiologists Warn of Critical Moment to Contain Monkeypox,” *PBS News Hour*, July 25, 2022, www.pbs.org/newshour/show/epidemiologists-warn-of-critical-moment-to-contain-monkeypox.
27. Ina Park and Dan Savage, “How Gay Men Saved Us from Mpox,” *New York Times*, April 16, 2023, www.nytimes.com/2023/04/16/opinion/gay-men-mpox.html.
28. Max Kozlov, “WHO [World Health Organization] May Soon End Mpox Emergency—but Outbreaks Rage in Africa,” *Nature*, February 10, 2023, www.nature.com/articles/d41586-023-00391-9. “Who is the ‘us’ that Dan Savage imagined is saved?” epidemiologist Joseph Osmundson wrote on Twitter/X. “Certainly not the Black same gender loving men in the US who died. Or the queer (and not queer) people in Nigeria who are still getting sick. Or queer people in Mexico where there is ZERO vaccine access.” Joseph Osmundson (@reluctantlyjoe), Twitter/X, April 16, 2023, https://twitter.com/reluctantlyjoe/status/1647645869078872065.
29. Annalisa Merelli, “90% of Mpox Deaths in the US Have Been Black Men,” Quartz, April 20, 2023, https://qz.com/mpox-deaths-disproportionately-black-men-cdc-report-1850338498.

Chronology

1. The chronology is based on the following sources: “Since AIDS, Boy’s Life a Court Battle,” *Indianapolis Star*, February 22, 1986, 11; “Ryan White Timeline,” *Kokomo Tribune*, September 24, 2006, C4; *NBC Nightly News*, August 26, 1985, record no. 545514, VTNA; ABC, *World News Tonight*, August 26, 1985, record no. 98027, VTNA; *NBC Nightly News*, February 21, 1986, record no. 548480, VTNA; White with Dworkin, *Weeding Out the Tears*; “The Ryan White HIV/AIDS Program: The Basics,” Kaiser Family Foundation, November 3, 2022, www.kff.org/hivaids/fact-sheet/the-ryan-white-hivaids-program-the-basics/.

BIBLIOGRAPHY

Archival Collections

ACT UP Oral History Project, actuporalhistory.org

The Ashes Action, dir. James Wentzy, AIDS Community Television (1992)

Tim Bailey's political funeral, footage by James Wentzy (July 1, 1993)

Mark Lowe Fisher's political funeral, footage by James Wentzy (November 2, 1992)

American Presidency Project, University of California, Santa Barbara, presidency.ucsb.edu

Archives of Women's Political Communication, Carrie Chapman Catt Center for Women and Politics, Iowa State University, Ames, awpc.cattcenter.iastate.edu

George H. W. Bush Presidential Library and Museum, College Station, TX

George H. W. Bush Presidential Records

Digital Library of Nonviolent Resistance, International Institute for Peace, Rutgers University, New Brunswick, NJ, nonviolence.rutgers.edu

Division of Rare and Manuscript Collections, Carl A. Kroch Library, Cornell University, Ithaca, NY

National LGBTQ Task Force Records (1973–2017) (also previously known as the National Gay Task Force Records and the National Gay and Lesbian Task Force Records)

Jesse Helms Center Archives, Wingate University, Wingate, NC

Jesse Helms Papers

Howard County Historical Society, Kokomo, IN

Ryan White Collection

Indiana State Archives, Indianapolis

Commissioners Files, Indiana State Board of Health

Indiana University Indianapolis Library, Digital Collections

Ryan White Letters

Indiana University Libraries, Bloomington

Moving Image Archive

Institute for Civic Leadership and Digital Mayoral Archives, University of Indianapolis, IN

L. Keith Bulen Collection

Manuscript and Archives Division, New York Public Library, New York City

Gran Fury Collection

Manuscript and Visual Collections Department, William Henry Smith Memorial Library, Indiana Historical Society, Indianapolis
ACLU of Indiana Records (1953–2013)
Michael Bohr Collection, Indy Pride Chris Gonzalez Library and Archives (ca. 1960s–2016)
Special Collections, University of California, San Francisco Libraries, Online Archive of California
Bobbi Campbell Diary
Special Collections Research Center, Gelman Library, George Washington University, Washington, DC
AIDS Action Foundation Records
Stanford Digital Repository, Stanford University Libraries, Stanford, CA, exhibits.stanford.edu/warhol
Andy Warhol Photography Collection
Vanderbilt Television News Archive, Vanderbilt University, Nashville, TN
Western Middle School Library Collection, Russiaville, IN
Personal Files of Ron Colby
Whitney Museum of American Art, New York City

Oral History Interviews

ACT UP Oral History Project, actuporalhistory.org
Joy Episalla, interview by Sarah Schulman, December 6, 2003
David Robinson, interview by Sarah Schulman, July 16, 2007
Howard County Historical Society, Kokomo, IN
Ryan White Oral History Project
Alan Adler, interview by Judy Lausch, March 23, 2009, object no. 2008.021.0002
Bev Ashcraft, interview by Judy Lausch, January 27, 2011, object no. 2011.065.0002
Rita Bagby, interview by Allen Safianow, January 20, 2011, object no. 2011.066.0002
Wanda Bilodeau, interview by Allen Safianow, June 7, 2011, object no. 2011.067.0002
Daniel W. Carter, interview by Allen Safianow, February 9, 2011, object no. 2011.068.0002
Ron Colby, interview by Diane Knight and Allen Safianow, May 24, 2011, object no. 2011.069.0002
Ken Ferries, interview by Allen Safianow, November 23, 2010, object no. 2011.070.0002
Cheryl Genovese, interview by Allen Safianow, October 14, 2010, object no. 2011.073.0002
Mitzie Johnson, interview by Diane Knight, June 30, 2011, object no. 2011.075.0002

Reverend Ruth Lawson, interview by Judy Lausch, February 17, 2011, object no. 2011.077.0002
Reverend Ray Probasco, interview by Allen Safianow, November 5, 2010, object no. 2011.080.0002
David Rosselot, interview by Diane Knight and Allen Safianow, October 13, 2011, object no. 2011.082.0002
John Wiles, interview by Judy Lausch, July 14, 2008, object no. 2008.020.0003

Visual Arts and the AIDS Epidemic: An Oral History Project, Smithsonian Archives of American Art, Smithsonian Institution, Washington, DC
Joy Episalla, interview by Cynthia Carr, February 23 and March 17, 2016

Periodicals and Digital Sources

ACT UP Historical Archive
The Advocate
The Advocate (Indiana Civil Liberties Union)
AIDS Weekly
Annals of Internal Medicine
Atlanta Constitution
The Atlantic
Bay Area Reporter
Boston Globe
Buzzfeed
Chicago Tribune
Clarksville (TN) Leaf-Chronicle
CNN.com
Daily Beast
Daily Hoosier
Daily Journal (IN)
Daily Times (Salisbury, MD)
Dame
Deconstructed podcast (*The Intercept*)
Emerge
Gay Community News (Boston)
GayLife (Chicago)
The Guardian
The Hill
Human Events
Indianapolis Monthly
Indianapolis News
Indianapolis Star
Indiana State Board of Health Bulletin
The Intercept
Kokomo (IN) Tribune
Life
Los Angeles Sentinel
Los Angeles Times
Morbidity and Mortality Weekly Report (*MMWR*)
National Public Radio
Nature
NBCNews.com
New Republic
Newsweek
New York Times
New York Times Magazine
Orange Coast Daily Pilot (CA)
Orlando Sentinel
Out/Look
Pensacola (FL) News Journal
People
Philadelphia Inquirer
POZ
Quartz
The Republic (IN)
Scientific American
Seattle Times
Star Tribune (MN)
STAT
Sun Sentinel (FL)
Tallahassee Democrat
Tampa Bay Times

Telegram & Gazette (MA)
Time
Towleroad
Twitter/X
USA Today
Village Voice
Wall Street Journal
Washington Post
Washington Times

Films and Televisual Sources

I Have AIDS: A Teenager's Story, 3–2–1 Contact: Extra. Children's Television Workshop, Public Broadcasting Service, 1988.

The Ryan White Story. Dir. John Herzfeld. ABC, 1989.

Books, Journal Articles, and Dissertations

Abramson, David Michael. "The Rules of Engagement: How Federal AIDS Policy Shaped Community Participation, and Was Shaped by It." PhD diss., Columbia University, 2005.

Andiman, Warren A. "Where Have All the 'AIDS Babies' Gone? A Historical Memoir of the Pediatric AIDS Epidemic in New Haven and Its Eventual Eradication." *Yale Journal of Biology and Medicine* 93, no. 4 (September 2020): 625–35.

Andriote, John-Manuel. *Victory Deferred: How AIDS Changed Gay Life in America.* Chicago: University of Chicago Press, 1999.

Arnesen, Eric. "Whiteness and the Historians' Imagination." *International Labor and Working-Class History* 60 (Fall 2001): 3–32.

Ayala, George, and Andrew Spieldenner. "HIV Is a Story First Written on the Bodies of Gay and Bisexual Men." *American Journal of Public Health* 111, no. 7 (July 2021): 1240–42.

Bayer, Ronald. "Gays and the Stigma of Bad Blood." *Hastings Center Report* 13, no. 2 (April 1983): 5–7.

———. "Science, Politics, and the End of the Lifelong Gay Blood Donor Ban." *Milbank Quarterly* 93, no. 2 (June 2015): 230–33.

Bell, Jonathan. "Between Private and Public: AIDS, Health Care Capitalism, and the Politics of Respectability in 1980s America." *Journal of American Studies* 54, no. 1 (February 2020): 159–83.

———, ed. *Beyond the Politics of the Closet: Gay Rights and the American State since the 1970s.* Philadelphia: University of Pennsylvania Press, 2020.

Bost, Darius. *Evidence of Being: The Black Gay Cultural Renaissance and the Politics of Violence.* Chicago: University of Chicago Press, 2018.

Brett, Jane. "The Experience of Disability from the Perspective of Parents of Children with Profound Impairment: Is It Time for an Alternative Model of Disability?" *Disability and Society* 17, no. 7 (2002): 825–43.

Brier, Jennifer. *Infectious Ideas: US Political Responses to the AIDS Crisis.* Chapel Hill: University of North Carolina Press, 2009.

———. "'Save Our Kids, Keep AIDS Out': Anti-AIDS Activism and the Legacy of Community Control in Queens, New York." *Journal of Social History* 39, no. 4 (Summer 2006): 965–87.

Briggs, Laura. *Somebody's Children: The Politics of Transracial and Transnational Adoption*. Durham, NC: Duke University Press, 2012.

Bryant, Anita. *The Anita Bryant Story: The Survival of Our Nation's Families and the Threat of Militant Homosexuality*. Old Tappan, NJ: Revell, 1977.

Bryan-Wilson, Julia. *Fray: Art and Textile Politics*. Chicago: University of Chicago Press, 2017.

Canaday, Margot. *Queer Career: Sexuality and Work in Modern America*. Princeton, NJ: Princeton University Press, 2023.

Carroll, Tamar W. *Mobilizing New York: AIDS, Antipoverty, and Feminist Activism*. Chapel Hill: University of North Carolina Press, 2015.

Centers for Disease Control and Prevention. *HIV Surveillance Supplemental Report* 26, no. 1 (2021). www.cdc.gov/hiv/pdf/library/reports/surveillance/cdc-hiv-surveillance-supplemental-report-vol-26-1.pdf.

Chávez, Karma R. *The Borders of AIDS: Race, Quarantine, and Resistance*. Seattle: University of Washington Press, 2021.

Cheng, Jih-Fei. "Cold Blood: HIV/AIDS and the Global Blood Biotechnology Industry." "The AIDS Crisis Is Not Over," edited by Emily K. Hobson and Dan Royles. Special issue, *Radical History Review*, no. 140 (May 2021): 143–50.

Cheng, Jih-Fei, Alexandra Juhasz, and Nishant Shahani. "Introduction." In Cheng, Juhasz, and Shahani, *AIDS and the Distribution of Crises*, 1–28.

———. "Preface." In Cheng, Juhasz, and Shahani, *AIDS and the Distribution of Crises*, xvii–xxvi.

———, eds. *AIDS and the Distribution of Crises*. Durham, NC: Duke University Press, 2020.

Cohen, Cathy J. *The Boundaries of Blackness: AIDS and the Breakdown of Black Politics*. Chicago: University of Chicago Press, 1999.

Cooper, Melinda. *Family Values: Between Neoliberalism and the New Social Conservatism*. New York: Zone Books, 2017.

Cram, E. "(Dis)locating Queer Citizenship: Imaging Rurality in Matthew Shepard's Memory." In Gray, Johnson, and Gilley, *Queering the Countryside*, 267–89.

Davidson, Michael. *Concerto for the Left Hand: Disability and the Defamiliar Body*. Ann Arbor: University of Michigan Press, 2008.

Des Jarlais, Don C., Thomas Kerr, Patrizia Carrieri, Jonathan Feelemyer, and Kamyar Arasteh. "HIV Infection among Persons Who Inject Drugs: Ending Old Epidemics and Addressing New Outbreaks." *AIDS* 30, no. 6 (March 2016): 815–26.

Des Jarlais, Don C., and Salaam Semaan. "HIV Prevention for Injecting Drug Users: The First 25 Years and Counting." *Psychosomatic Medicine* 70, no. 5 (June 2008): 606–11.

"Dispatches on the Globalizations of AIDS: A Dialogue between Theodore (Ted)

Kerr, Catherine Yuk-ping Lo, Ian Bradley-Perrin, Sarah Schulman, and Eric A. Stanley, with an Introduction by Nishant Shahani." In Cheng, Juhasz, and Shahani, *AIDS and the Distribution of Crises*, 29–59.

Donovan, Mark C. "The Problem with Making AIDS Comfortable: Federal Policy Making and the Rhetoric of Innocence." *Journal of Homosexuality* 32, nos. 3–4 (1997): 115–44.

Du Bois, W. E. B. *Black Reconstruction in America, 1860–1880*. 1935. Reprint, New York: Free Press, 1998.

Egan, Timothy. *A Fever in the Heartland: The Ku Klux Klan's Plot to Take Over America, and the Woman Who Stopped Them*. New York: Viking, 2023.

Epstein, Steven. *Impure Science: AIDS, Activism, and the Politics of Knowledge*. Berkeley: University of California Press, 1996.

Faria, Nuno R., et al. "The Early Spread and Epidemic Ignition of HIV-1 in Human Populations." *Science* 346 (October 2014): 56–61.

Farmer, Paul. *AIDS and Accusation: Haiti and the Geography of Blame*. Berkeley: University of California Press, 2006.

Fields, Barbara J. "Whiteness, Racism, and Identity." *International Labor and Working-Class History* 60 (Fall 2001): 48–56.

Fink, Marty. *Forget Burial: HIV Kinship, Disability, and Queer/Trans Narratives of Care*. New Brunswick, NJ: Rutgers University Press, 2020.

Fleegler, Robert L. *Brutal Campaign: How the 1988 Election Set the Stage for Twenty-First-Century American Politics*. Chapel Hill: University of North Carolina Press, 2023.

Frank, Gillian. "'The Civil Rights of Parents': Race and Conservative Politics in Anita Bryant's Campaign against Gay Rights in 1970s Florida." *Journal of the History of Sexuality* 22, no. 1 (2013): 126–60.

Fumento, Michael. *The Myth of Heterosexual AIDS: How a Tragedy Has Been Distorted by the Media and Partisan Politics*. New York: Regnery Gateway, 1990.

Ganz, John. *When the Clock Broke: Con Men, Conspiracists, and How America Cracked Up in the Early 1990s*. New York: Farrar, Straus and Giroux, 2024.

Garretson, Jeremiah J. *The Path to Gay Rights: How Activism and Coming Out Changed Public Opinion*. New York: New York University Press, 2018.

Gomer, Justin. *White Balance: How Hollywood Shaped Colorblind Ideology and Undermined Civil Rights*. Chapel Hill: University of North Carolina Press, 2020.

Gordon, Linda. *The Second Coming of the KKK: The Ku Klux Klan of the 1920s and the American Political Tradition*. New York: Liveright, 2017.

Gould, Deborah B. *Moving Politics: Emotion and ACT UP's Fight against AIDS*. Chicago: University of Chicago Press, 2009.

Gray, Mary L., Colin R. Johnson, and Brian J. Gilley, eds. *Queering the Countryside: New Frontiers in Rural Queer Studies*. New York: New York University Press, 2016.

Grmek, Mirko D. *History of AIDS: Emergence and Origin of a Modern Pandemic*. Princeton, NJ: Princeton University Press, 1990.

Halperin, David M., and Trevor Hoppe, eds. *The War on Sex*. Durham, NC: Duke University Press, 2017.

Hammonds, Evelynn. "Race, Sex, AIDS: The Construction of 'Other.'" *Radical America* 20 (November–December 1987): 28–38.

Harsono, Dini, Carol L. Galletly, Elaine O'Keefe, and Zita Lazzarini. "Criminalization of HIV Exposure: A Review of Empirical Studies in the United States." *AIDS and Behavior* 21, no. 1 (January 2017): 27–50.

Hartman, Andrew. *A War for the Soul of America: A History of the Culture Wars*. Chicago: University of Chicago Press, 2015.

Hemmer, Nicole. *Partisans: The Conservative Revolutionaries Who Remade American Politics in the 1990s*. New York: Basic Books, 2022.

Herring, Scott. *Another Country: Queer Anti-Urbanism*. New York: New York University Press, 2010.

Hobson, Emily K. *Lavender and Red: Liberation and Solidarity in the Gay and Lesbian Left*. Berkeley: University of California Press, 2016.

Hobson, Emily K., and Dan Royles, eds. "The AIDS Crisis Is Not Over." Special issue, *Radical History Review*, no. 140 (May 2021).

Hobson, Emily K., and Dan Royles. "Editors' Introduction." In "The AIDS Crisis Is Not Over." Special issue, *Radical History Review*, no. 140 (May 2021): 1–8.

Hogan, Katie. *Women Take Care: Gender, Race, and the Culture of AIDS*. Ithaca, NY: Cornell University Press, 2001.

Hoppe, Trevor. *Punishing Disease: HIV and the Criminalization of Sickness*. Berkeley: University of California Press, 2017.

HoSang, Daniel Martinez. *Racial Propositions: Ballot Initiatives and the Making of Postwar California*. Berkeley: University of California Press, 2010.

Howard, John. *Men Like That: A Southern Queer History*. Chicago: University of Chicago Press, 1999.

Hubbs, Nadine. *Rednecks, Queers, and Country Music*. Berkeley: University of California Press, 2014.

Ignatiev, Noel. *How the Irish Became White*. New York: Routledge, 1995.

Institute of Medicine, Division of Health Promotion and Disease Prevention, Committee to Study HIV Transmission through Blood and Blood Products. *HIV and the Blood Supply: An Analysis of Crisis Decisionmaking*. Washington, DC: National Academy Press, 1995.

"Interchange: HIV/AIDS and US History." *Journal of American History* 104, no. 2 (September 2017): 431–60.

Jacobson, Matthew Frye. *Whiteness of a Different Color: European Immigrants and the Alchemy of Race*. Cambridge, MA: Harvard University Press, 1998.

John, Elton. *Love Is the Cure: On Life, Loss, and the End of AIDS*. New York: Back Bay, 2012.

Johnson, Colin R. *Just Queer Folks: Gender and Sexuality in Rural America*. Philadelphia: Temple University Press, 2013.

Johnson, E. Patrick. *Sweet Tea: Black Gay Men of the South*. Chapel Hill: University of North Carolina Press, 2008.

Johnson, Walter. *The Broken Heart of America: St. Louis and the Violent History of the United States*. New York: Basic Books, 2020.

Juhasz, Alexandra, and Theodore Kerr. *We Are Having This Conversation Now: The Times of AIDS Cultural Production*. Durham, NC: Duke University Press, 2022.

Kerr, Theodore. "How to Live with a Virus." *QED: A Journal in GLBTQ Worldmaking* 7, no. 3 (Fall 2020): 109–16.

King, Edward. *Safety in Numbers: Safer Sex and Gay Men*. New York: Routledge, 1994.

Kitzinger, Celia, and Elizabeth Peel. "The De-gaying and Re-gaying of AIDS: Contested Homophobias in Lesbian and Gay Awareness Training." *Discourse and Society* 16, no. 2 (March 2005): 173–97.

Kohler-Hausmann, Julilly. *Getting Tough: Welfare and Imprisonment in 1970s America*. Princeton, NJ: Princeton University Press, 2017.

Kolchin, Peter. "Whiteness Studies: The New History of Race in America." *Journal of American History* 89, no. 1 (June 2002): 154–73.

Lassiter, Matthew D., and Joseph Crespino, eds. *The Myth of Southern Exceptionalism*. New York: Oxford University Press, 2010.

Levine, Debra. "How to Do Things with Dead Bodies." *Emisférica* 6, no. 1 (Summer 2009). https://hemisphericinstitute.org/en/emisferica-61/6-1-essays/how-to-do-things-with-dead-bodies.html.

Lichtenstein, Nelson, and Judith Stein. *A Fabulous Failure: The Clinton Presidency and the Transformation of American Capitalism*. Princeton, NJ: Princeton University Press, 2023.

Lipsitz, George. *The Possessive Investment in Whiteness: How White People Profit from Identity Politics*. Philadelphia: Temple University Press, 1998.

Lowery, Jack. *It Was Vulgar and It Was Beautiful: How AIDS Activists Used Art to Fight a Pandemic*. New York: Bold Type Books, 2022.

Macek, Steve. *Urban Nightmares: The Media, the Right, and the Moral Panic over the City*. Minneapolis: University of Minnesota Press, 2006.

Mackenzie, Sonja. *Structural Intimacies: Sexual Stories in the Black AIDS Epidemic*. New Brunswick, NJ: Rutgers University Press, 2013.

Madison, James H. *The Ku Klux Klan in the Heartland*. Bloomington: Indiana University Press, 2020.

Manalansan, Martin F., Chantal Nadeau, Richard T. Rodriguez, and Siobham B. Somerville, eds. "Queering the Middle: Race, Region, and a Queer Midwest." Special issue, *GLQ: A Journal of Lesbian and Gay Studies* 20, nos. 1–2 (Spring 2014).

McKay, Richard A. *Patient Zero and the Making of the AIDS Epidemic*. Chicago: University of Chicago Press, 2017.

———. "'Patient Zero': The Absence of a Patient's View of the Early North American AIDS Epidemic." *Bulletin of the History of Medicine* 88, no. 1 (Spring 2014): 161–94.

Meeropol, Michael. *Surrender: How the Clinton Administration Completed the Reagan Revolution*. Ann Arbor: University of Michigan Press, 1998.

Moore, Leonard J. *Citizen Klansmen: The Ku Klux Klan in Indiana, 1921–1928*. Chapel Hill: University of North Carolina Press, 1991.

Mumford, Kevin. *Not Straight, Not White: Black Gay Men from the March on Washington to the AIDS Crisis*. Chapel Hill: University of North Carolina Press, 2016.

Murch, Donna. "Who's to Blame for Mass Incarceration?" *Boston Review*, October 16, 2015. www.bostonreview.net/articles/donna-murch-michael-javen-fortner-black-silent-majority/.

Murphy, Timothy F. "No Time for an AIDS Backlash." *Hastings Center Report* 21, no. 2 (March–April 1991): 7–11.

Nicholas, Stephen W., and Elaine J. Abrams. "Boarder Babies with AIDS in Harlem: Lessons in Applied Public Health." *American Journal of Public Health* 92, no. 2 (February 2002): 163–65.

O'Daniel, Alyson. *Holding On: African American Women Surviving HIV/AIDS*. Lincoln: University of Nebraska Press, 2016.

Painter, Nell Irvin. *The History of White People*. New York: W. W. Norton, 2010.

Paone, Denise, Don C. Des Jarlais, Stephanie Caloir, Patricia Freidmann, and Immanuel Ness. "New York City Syringe Exchange: An Overview." *Proceedings Workshop on Needle Exchange and Bleach Distribution Programs*. Washington, DC: National Academies Press, 1994.

Passanante Elman, Julie. *Chronic Youth: Disability, Sexuality, and US Media Cultures of Rehabilitation*. New York: New York University Press, 2014.

Patton, Cindy. *Fatal Advice: How Safe-Sex Education Went Wrong*. Durham, NC: Duke University Press, 1996.

———. "Fear of AIDS: The Erotics of Innocence and Ingenuity." *American Imago* 49, no. 3 (Fall 1992): 323–41.

———. "Foreword." In Cheng, Juhasz, and Shahani, *AIDS and the Distribution of Crises*, vii–xvi.

———. *Last Served? Gendering the HIV Pandemic*. Bristol, PA: Taylor and Francis, 1994.

Pemberton, Stephen. *The Bleeding Disease: Hemophilia and the Unintended Consequences of Medical Progress*. Baltimore: Johns Hopkins University Press, 2011.

———. "The Curious Case of the 'Professional Hemophiliac': Medicine, Disability, and the Contested Value of Normality in the United States, 1940–2010." In *Disability Histories*, edited by Susan Burch and Michael Rembis, 237–57. Urbana: University of Illinois Press, 2014.

Pépin, Jacques. *The Origins of AIDS*. Rev. and updated ed. New York: Cambridge University Press, 2021.

Peters, Philip J., et al. "HIV Infection Linked to Injection Use of Oxymorphone in Indiana, 2014–2015." *New England Journal of Medicine* 375 (July 21, 2016): 229–39.

Petro, Anthony M. *After the Wrath of God: AIDS, Sexuality, and American Religion*. New York: Oxford University Press, 2015.

Phillips-Fein, Kim. *Fear City: New York's Fiscal Crisis and the Rise of Austerity Politics*. New York: Metropolitan Books, 2017.

Poindexter, Cynthia Cannon. "Promises in the Plague: Passage of the Ryan White Comprehensive AIDS Resources Emergency Act as a Case Study for Legislative Action." *Health and Social Work* 24, no. 1 (February 1999): 35–41.

Price, Nelson. *The Quiet Hero: A Life of Ryan White*. Indianapolis: Indiana Historical Society Press, 2015.

Reichard, Ruth. *Blood and Steel: Ryan White, the AIDS Crisis, and Deindustrialization in Kokomo, Indiana*. Jefferson, NC: McFarland, 2021.

Resnik, Susan. *Blood Saga: Hemophilia, AIDS, and the Survival of a Community*. Updated ed. Berkeley: University of California Press, 1999.

Roediger, David R. *The Wages of Whiteness: Race and the Making of the American Working Class*. New York: Verso, 1991.

Royles, Dan. "HIV/AIDS in the United States." In *Global Encyclopedia of Lesbian, Gay, Bisexual, Transgender, and Queer (LGBTQ) History*, edited by Howard Chiang, 734–42. Farmington Hills, MI: Gale, 2019.

———. "Love and Rage." *Nursing Clio* (blog), March 9, 2017. https://nursingclio.org/2017/03/09/love-and-rage/.

———. *To Make the Wounded Whole: The African American Struggle against HIV/AIDS*. Chapel Hill: University of North Carolina Press, 2020.

Schulman, Sarah. *Let the Record Show: A Political History of ACT UP New York, 1987–1993*. New York: Farrar, Straus and Giroux, 2021.

Sheridan, Thomas F. *Helping the Good Do Better: How a White Hat Lobbyist Advocates for Social Change*. New York: Twelve Books, 2019.

Shilts, Randy. *And the Band Played On: Politics, People, and the AIDS Epidemic*. New York: St. Martin's Press, 1987.

Siplon, Patricia D. *AIDS and the Policy Struggle in the United States*. Washington, DC: Georgetown University Press, 2002.

———. "Washington's Response to the AIDS Epidemic: The Ryan White CARE Act." *Policy Studies Journal* 27, no. 4 (1999): 796–808.

Stewart-Winter, Timothy. *Queer Clout: Chicago and the Rise of Gay Politics*. Philadelphia: University of Pennsylvania Press, 2016.

Sturken, Marita. *Tangled Memories: The Vietnam War, the AIDS Epidemic, and the Politics of Remembering*. Berkeley: University of California Press, 1997.

Taylor-Brown, Susan. "'Women Don't Get AIDS: They Just Die from It.'" *Affilia: Journal of Women and Social Work* 7, no. 4 (Winter 1992): 96–98.

Testa, Nino. "'If You Are Reading It, I Am Dead': Activism, Local History, and the AIDS Quilt." *Public Historian* 44, no. 3 (August 2022): 24–57.

Thrasher, Steven W. *The Viral Underclass: The Human Toll When Inequality and Disease Collide*. New York: Celadon Books, 2022.

Tomso, Gregory. "HIV Monsters: Gay Men, Criminal Law, and the New Political Economy of HIV." In Halperin and Hoppe, *The War on Sex*, 353–77.

Treichler, Paula A. *How to Have Theory in an Epidemic: Cultural Chronicles of AIDS*. Durham, NC: Duke University Press, 1999.

Vaid, Urvashi. *Virtual Equality: The Mainstreaming of Gay and Lesbian Liberation*. New York: Anchor Books, 1995.

Vider, Stephen. *The Queerness of Home: Gender, Sexuality, and the Politics of Domesticity after World War II*. Chicago: University of Chicago Press, 2021.

Von Eschen, Penny. *Paradoxes of Nostalgia: Cold War Triumphalism and Global Disorder since 1989*. Durham, NC: Duke University Press, 2022.

Warner, Michael. *The Trouble with Normal: Sex, Politics, and the Ethics of Queer Life*. New York: Free Press, 1999.

Watkins-Hayes, Celeste. *Remaking a Life: How Women Living with HIV/AIDS Confront Inequality*. Berkeley: University of California Press, 2019.

Watney, Simon. *Policing Desire: Pornography, AIDS, and the Media*. Minneapolis: University of Minnesota Press, 1987.

White, Jeanne, with Susan Dworkin. *Weeding Out the Tears: A Mother's Story of Love, Loss, and Renewal*. New York: Avon Books, 1997.

White, Ryan, and Ann Marie Cunningham. *Ryan White: My Own Story*. New York: Berkley Publishing, 1991.

Wojnarowicz, David. *Close to the Knives: A Memoir of Disintegration*. New York: Vintage, 1991.

Wright, Joe. "Only Your Calamity: The Beginnings of Activism by and for People with AIDS." *American Journal of Public Health* 103, no. 10 (October 2013): 1788–98.

Yingling, Thomas E. *AIDS and the National Body*. Edited and with an introduction by Robyn Wiegman. Durham, NC: Duke University Press, 1997.

INDEX